"I suffered from headache for over 20 years and attended Dr Kanji in 2012. I sought him out as he studied thousands of articles on headache and migraine in his PhD. He found out my neck was causing my pain and explained how this contributed to headache.

"My headache, migraine and neck pain symptoms are now gone. I no longer need to take the countless medications, and my head is clear for the first time in decades. I was given the advice in this book and have never looked back. Thank you Dr Kanji for trying to solve the problem rather than place a band aid on it."

P N Wellington

This book is dedicated to my wife Sathna, my children Ataya, Keelan and Jessica for their patience and support.

To my late father, Kanji, and mother Laxmi for their love and perseverance.

To my patients, and colleagues.

And to Professor Nikolai Bogduk, Associate Professor Rachel Page and the late Dr Jayantilal Govind who inspired me to continue learning.

Giresh Kanji

Fix your Neck pain Headache & Migraine

DR GIRESH KANJI

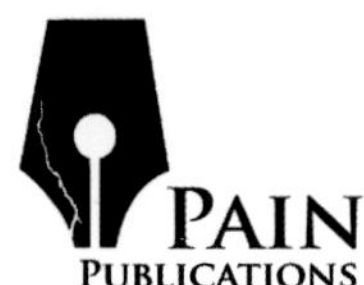

First published in 2015 by Pain Publications,
Level 2, 354 Lambton Quay, Wellington, New Zealand

National Library of New Zealand Cataloguing-in-Publication Data

Kanji, Giresh, 1966-
Fix Your Neck Pain Headache & Migraine / author: Dr Giresh Kanji.
Includes bibliographical references.
ISBN 978-0-473-32281-6
1. Neck pain. 2. Neck pain—Treatment. 3. Headache—Popular works.
4. Migraine—Popular works. I. Title.
617.5306—dc 23

Editor: Max Rashbrooke
Cover design: Preehya Patel/Selena Henry/Sejal Bhikha
Illustrator: Preehya Patel, Selena Henry, Sejal Bhikha
Printed by Printlink, Wellington, New Zealand

www.painpublications.com

About the author

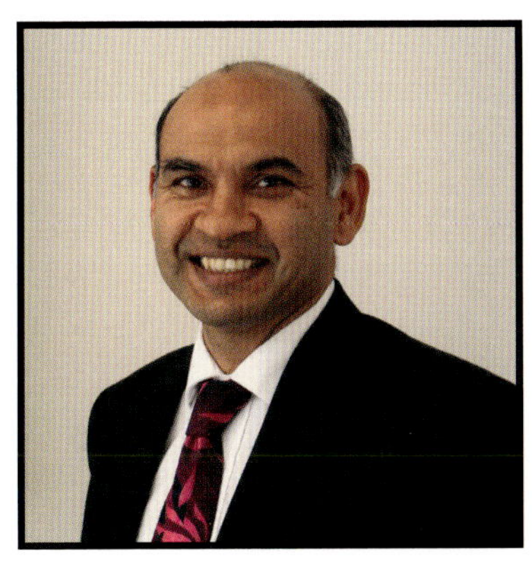

Dr Giresh Kanji was born in Wellington, New Zealand, and educated at Wellington College, Otago Medical School and Massey University. He finished a PhD investigating chronic pain in 2013. He has worked as a medical doctor since 1990 and has been treating chronic pain patients in Wellington since 1995. He set up the Sports and Pain Clinic in Wellington in 2011 to treat patients and perform research. An Auckland branch was opened in 2015 to allow multicentre clinical trials to be performed. After completion of his studies, he founded the New Zealand Pain Foundation to carry out research into chronic pain disorders. He is currently supervising research on back pain, neck pain and depression. In 2014 he was appointed the editor of the *Australasian Musculoskeletal Medicine Journal*. This book is Dr Kanji's second book and follows *Fix Your Back*, which is in its third print and has sold nearly 10,000 copies. Giresh is married with three children.

CONTENTS

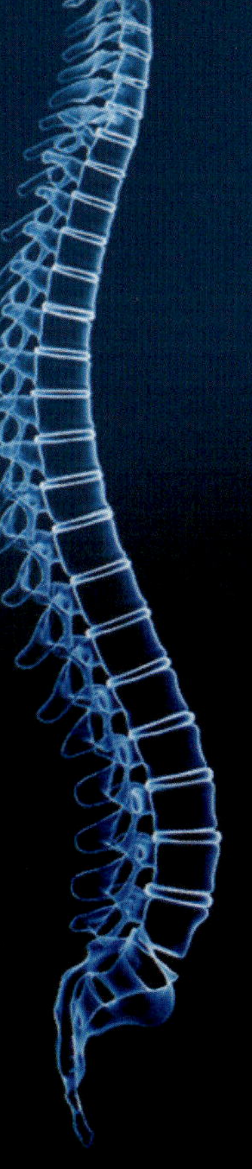

Contents

CONTENTS

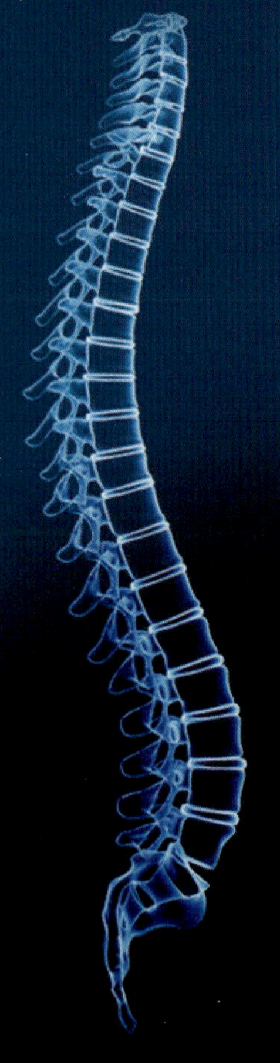

Introduction

I am very pleased to have finished this book on neck pain, headache and migraine over the past two years. After completing my PhD which focused on headache and migraine, I wanted to collate this together with what I have learned from patients over the past few decades in a book. It is my hope that this book will be an easy to understand way to help people fix their own neck pain, headache and migraine. For those of you who have not read my first book *Fix Your Back* I have copied some of the introduction from this book to give you some background on my work.

I started working full time in pain medicine over ten years ago and recall going to work with a feeling of dread. What was I going to do to help these patients? Prescribe medication that never seemed to cure the suffering and often caused side effects? I was no longer happy prescribing medications without trying to understand the cause of people's pain. I decided to investigate why people developed pain and how to reduce it.

After years of treating chronic pain patients, I noticed that pain spreads and intensifies with time, making it difficult to diagnose its source. Often the patient's pain may no longer be at the site of injury and the diagnosis becomes blurred for both the patient and the health professional.

Chronic lower back pain is a significant worldwide medical puzzle with reportedly no cause found in up to 85% of cases[1]*. So what do you do when you cannot find the cause and treat pain? Call in the psychologist and psychiatrist to help people cope with their symptoms? I feel that the medical profession has failed these patients. Many patients do not understand why they are seeking psychological help, often feeling that the doctor thinks the problem is in their head! After seeing numerous specialists without any answers, a patient may believe this to be true.*

My journey into examining the chronic pain puzzle started in earnest back in July 2005. I was researching a presentation on referred pain for the New Zealand Association of Musculoskeletal Medicine conference in Dunedin, New Zealand. I became curious about where people's pain comes from, how it spreads and amplifies, and why almost everyone with chronic pain develops problems such as insomnia, anxiety, depression and mental irritability.

I became fascinated and spent several years examining scientific literature to try and solve the puzzle of pain. I read books on biochemistry, neurophysiology, neurology, and the sympathetic nervous system (stress nervous system) and made countless computer searches on various topics. I would wake between four and five a.m. and read and write for several hours before work. This habit remained for many years as the puzzle of pain started unfolding. During this time I completed two business degrees and read many books on critical thinking. The biggest lesson I learned was to keep asking why until a satisfactory answer is found, otherwise you only get half-truths and half-cures.

My journey culminated in spending five years working towards a PhD thesis. I created a model to explain why pain amplifies and spreads throughout the body after examining over 600 scientific papers and dozens of books.

I wanted to find the cause of people's pain and reduce their pain scores to zero (zero being no pain, ten being the worst pain imaginable). If a patient's pain could not be eliminated I hoped to find its cause, as the most frustrating thing for patients is not knowing what is causing their pain. Furthermore, if the source of pain is known, then treatment can be targeted at the problem. If no treatment is available, then time and money need not be wasted on therapy that may not help.

Although I have managed my patients' chronic pain conditions for over 20 years I did not recognise my own symptoms. I experienced pins and needles and numbness in both arms for many years, especially when I was sleeping. I changed my pillow at least a dozen times to try to alleviate the symptoms.

I also recall experiencing neck pain at times, during my PhD, when sitting at the computer for long periods. Finally, in 2012, I obtained an MRI scan that showed me what was wrong with my neck and allowed me to treat myself to reduce my symptoms, which have over the past 12 months, almost completely gone. I have shared my story and scans in Chapter 1.

This book follows my first publication, *Fix Your Back*, and looks at the second most common source of pain (after the back) – the neck. I have included headache and migraine in this book as treating neck pain is integral to the management of those conditions. *Fix Your Neck Headache & Migraine* describes the structures in the neck that cause pain, their contributions to headaches, and how to unravel the mysteries of migraine.

I hope to reach people who are suffering from neck pain, headache and migraine, to provide some explanation of their symptoms, outline investigations that can be performed, and describe possible treatment options. My thanks go out to all the patients who have allowed their stories to appear in this book. All names have been changed so patients cannot be identified.

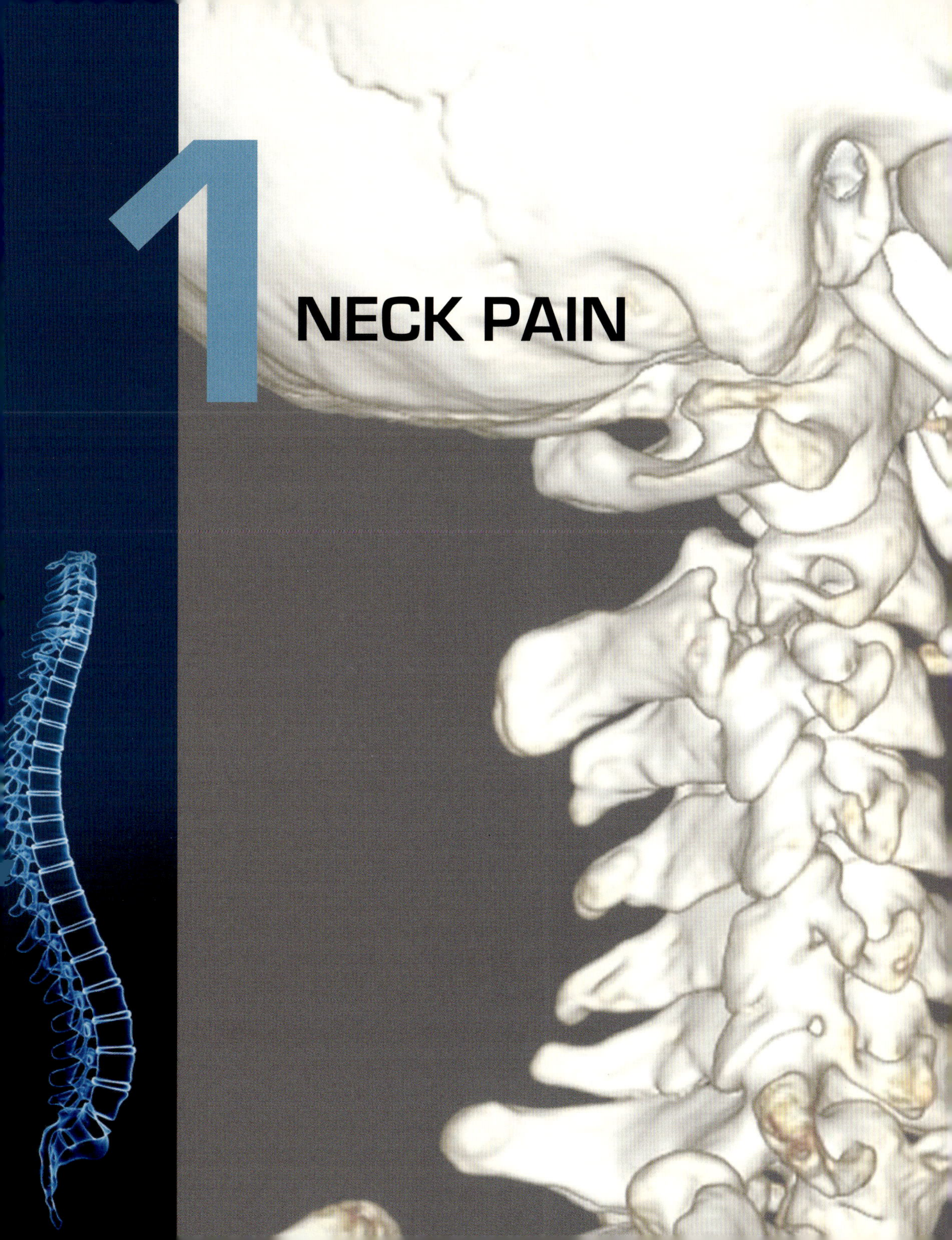

1 NECK PAIN

Neck pain

After back pain, neck pain is the most frequent musculoskeletal cause of medical consultations worldwide. Fortunately, a new episode of neck pain usually resolves within a few days or weeks. Approximately two-thirds of the population experience neck pain at some time in their lives, and most often neck pain peaks at middle age. Surveys have shown that 25% of the population are experiencing neck pain at any one time. But neck pain does not always subside, and people often experience frequent episodes throughout the year. In one survey, 60% of people with neck pain still experienced it a year later.

Unfortunately, when neck pain continues for months or years, you are rarely advised what is causing it. Sometimes stress, tight muscles, poor posture, not enough exercise, lack of vitamins or minerals, or a joint out of place are all blamed as the cause of your symptoms. Furthermore, investigations of the neck do not tell the whole story, leaving both you and the treatment provider in the dark. Once you have been involved in an accident such as a fall or whiplash, structures can become damaged, but conventional X-rays often show nothing. An autopsy study of 21 people who had sustained fatal head and neck injuries from motor vehicle accidents revealed that 198 lesions were missed on X-rays.[1] These included fractures, disc injuries, ligament and muscle tears, and facet joint injuries.

Most people with neck pain experience broken sleep, often trying several different pillows to find the right position to avoid pain. Some struggle to get to sleep because they cannot find a comfortable position, while others wake frequently with neck pain and stiffness. Sleep disturbance adds to the misery of neck pain and helps to activate stress-related symptoms like insomnia, anxiety, depression and irritability.

While neck pain is a burden to individuals, it is also a significant and costly problem in Western societies. Every year the number of people who develop long-term neck pain increases. Some cannot return to work and the monetary cost of treatment mounts with each passing year. The workers' compensation available in the West has placed financial burdens on both the suffering individual and society at large. However, the money received by those on workers' compensation rarely makes up for the immense suffering they feel.

A logical approach to treating neck pain is to perform tests that will exclude, one after another, the structures that may be causing pain, using simple treatments initially, then progressing to more invasive treatments. Any structure with a nerve supply is capable of causing pain, including ligaments, tendons, muscles, bones, discs and joints.

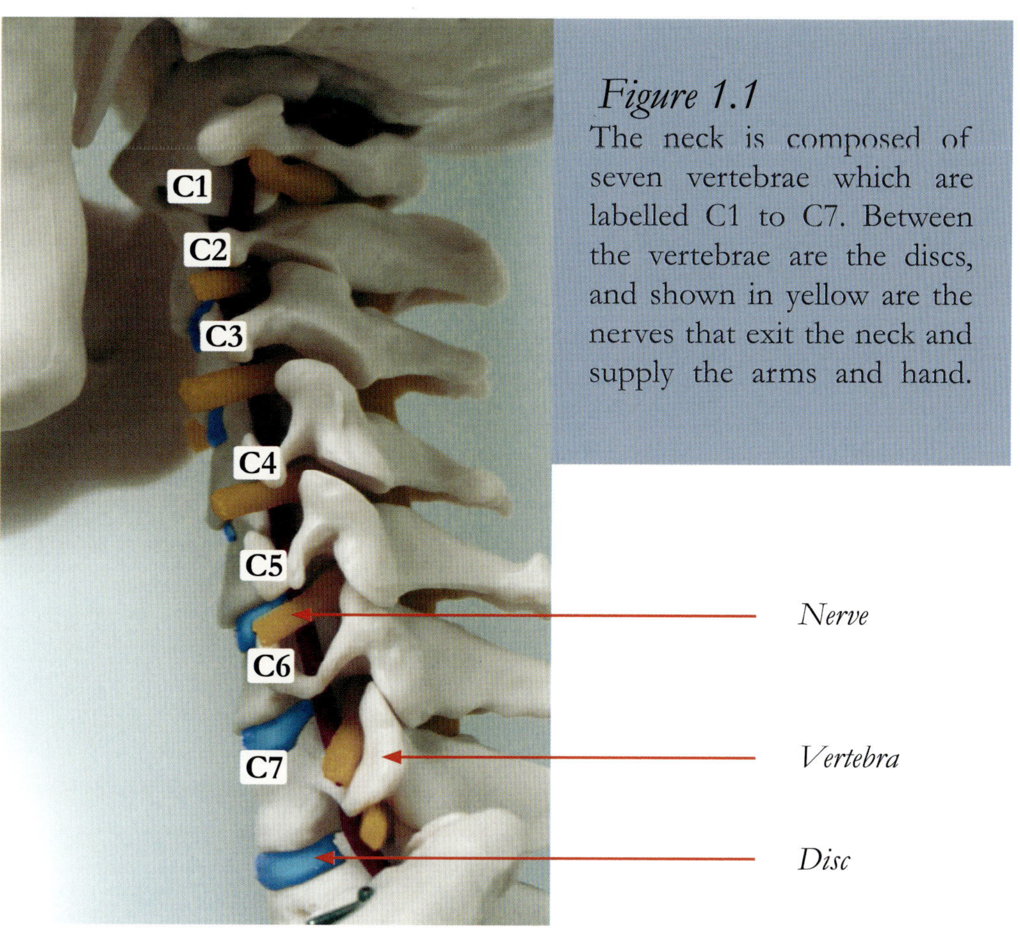

Figure 1.1
The neck is composed of seven vertebrae which are labelled C1 to C7. Between the vertebrae are the discs, and shown in yellow are the nerves that exit the neck and supply the arms and hand.

For practical purposes, the tissues that cause pain are best separated into soft tissues (ligaments, muscles, tendons and discs) and hard tissues (bone and facet joints). When treatment is applied to the soft tissues of the neck, if someone gets 100% relief of their pain then it is reasonable to conclude that their pain was caused by soft tissues. Those improving by 50% will have some contribution of pain from their soft tissues, but other deeper structures are also likely to be contributing to their pain.

CASE STUDY: *Giresh Kanji*

For many years I experienced intermittent neck pain. This was at its worst when I was finishing my PhD as it required many hours of reading and writing, often looking at a computer screen and reading medical papers. Night time was the worst time, when I would wake with my whole arm feeling hollow and empty. I would shift around and feeling would return to the arm. I would also experience pins and needles in my fingers when sleeping. I had muscle spasm around my neck and jaw region. Some nights I would wake in the middle of the night feeling like I had been choking. I never slept well, and woke tired. Over the years I tried several pillows, some very expensive, to try to reduce the night symptoms. I did not really know the cause of my symptoms. I often thought it was due to a hard bed, but even after changing the bed there was no improvement. Sometimes I wore a soft collar at night which helped me sleep but was uncomfortable, especially in summer due to the heat it generated. I enjoyed road cycling and participated in the Lake Taupo Cycle Challenge, the thing that hurt the most as I was heading to the finish line was my neck. As well as neck pain, I also started noticing a feeling of inco-ordination when running, as if my feet were slapping down all the time. I had been a runner for years and did not take any notice of this symptom initially. In 2012 an MRI scan of my neck was performed. This showed disc narrowing and compression of the spinal cord. In a way I was relieved to find the cause of my symptoms. When looking back the single biggest trauma I had sustained was in a motor vehicle accident in which I fractured my leg and spent nine weeks in leg traction at Wellington Hospital. I suspect this was the first incident that may have caused disc damage and over the next several decades the disc narrowed, creating the changes visible on the scan. I started changing my posture to reduce pressure on my discs, wearing a soft collar when traveling in a plane, and using traction devices and exercises as described in Chapter 5. Over the next six months my symptoms reduced significantly, to the point where now I only experience symptoms once every few months. The pins and needles and hollow feelings in my arms has been absent for many months. I have returned to running and my co-ordination when running has improved. I am enjoying much better sleep and the muscle spasm around the neck and jaw has reduced. I am back to dreaming most nights. I was worried that I would require an operation to reduce the pressure on my spinal cord so am very pleased I was able to manage my symptoms.

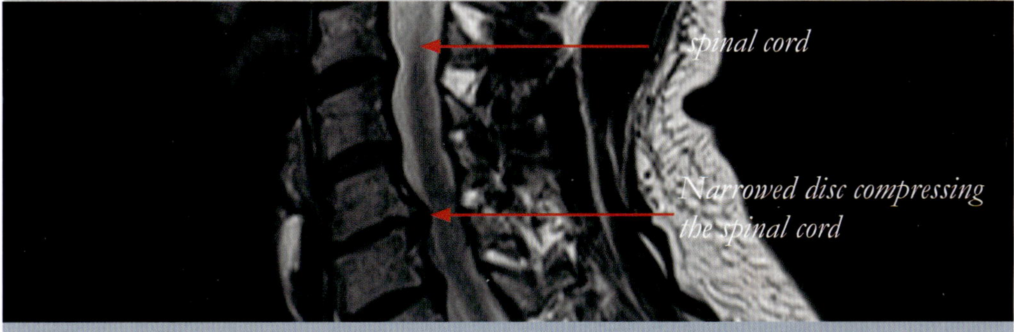

Figure 1.2

The MRI scan shows narrowing of the discs at C5/6 and 6/7 with disc bulging posteriorly touching the spinal cord.

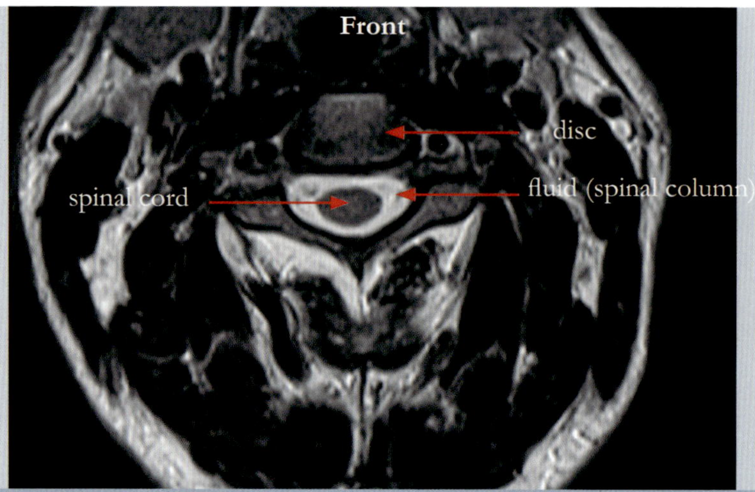

Figure 1.3
A cross-section of the neck with fluid (in white) between the disc and spinal cord.

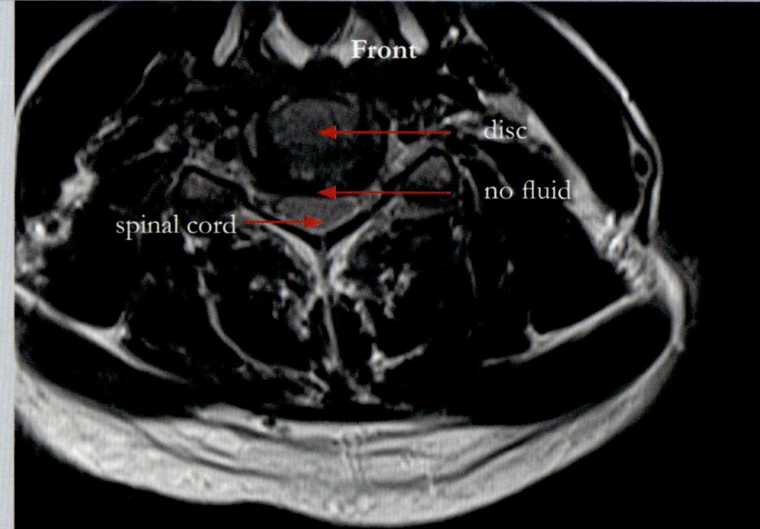

Figure 1.4
An MRI scan cross-section showing no space between the disc and the spinal cord. The disc is pressing against the spinal cord at this level.

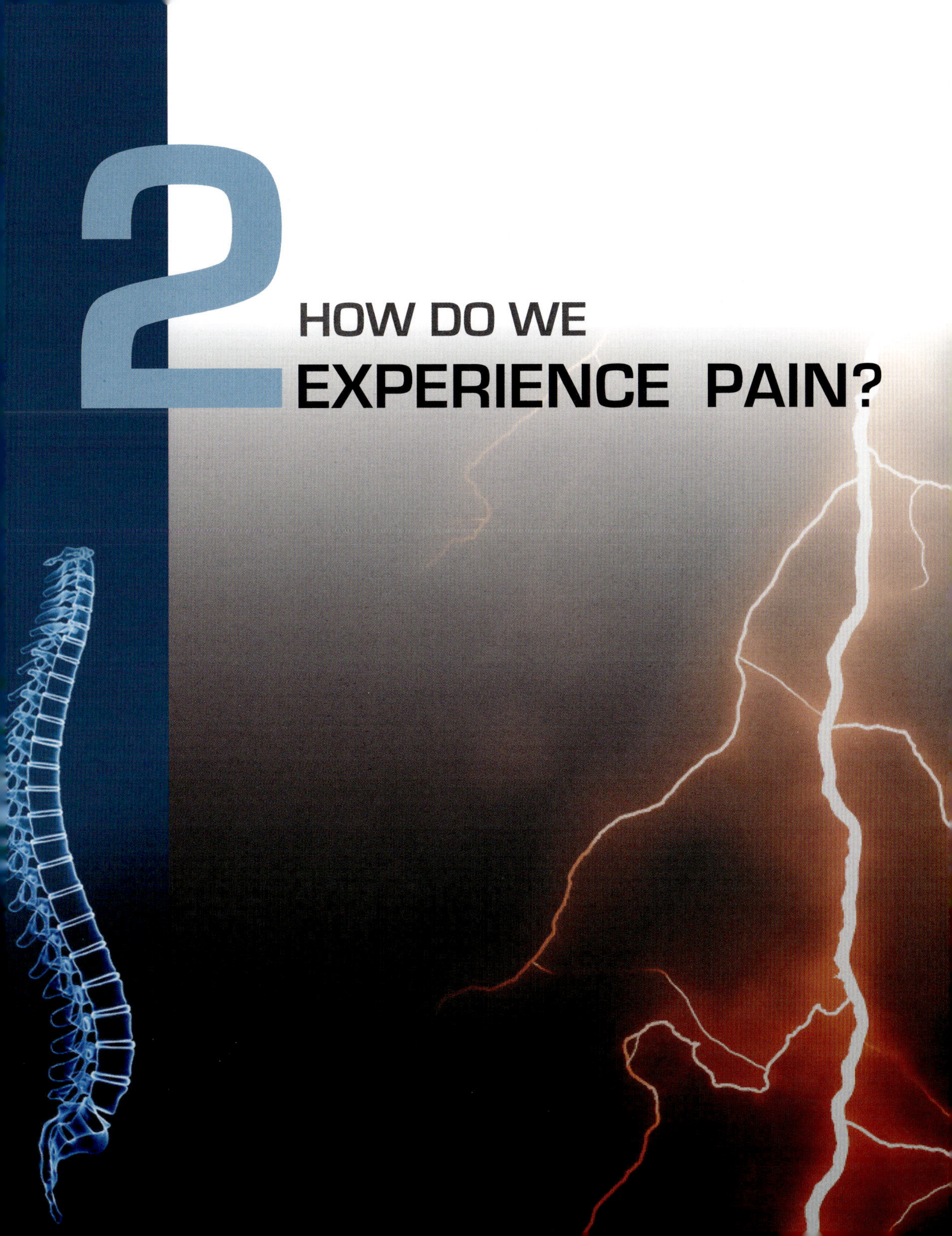

2 HOW DO WE EXPERIENCE PAIN?

What is pain?

Pain can be defined as an unpleasant sensory and emotional experience. But how is it produced and how does the brain know a part of the body has been injured? Receptors are present in the skin, muscles, joints, ligaments, tendons and discs, and they detect pressure, stretch, chemicals, heat and pain. Once a receptor is activated, an electrical spark is generated and transmitted along nerves to the brain (Figure 2.1), like electricity conducting through copper wires. Without this conduction, there is no pain.

When you feel a pinprick, the skin damage is sensed by pain and pressure receptors; this creates an electrical spark that travels through switches in the spinal cord and brain, and is interpreted as pain. The brain forms a picture of the site of pain and its intensity, and even sends messages to the emotional centres of the brain.

Structures in the body, such as discs and cartilage, are designed to reduce pressure on the bones. Once these are damaged, pressure falls onto the bones and discs, and sensors that lie within the bones and discs create electrical sparks that can be experienced as pain.

The level of pain experienced depends on several factors.

First, the extent of disc damage. The greater the disc damage, the less it is able to absorb pressure, resulting in increased pain, because more bony receptors are creating electrical sparks.

Second, the level of pain is determined by the intensity and time a force is applied to the disc. A large force acting for a short time is the same as a small force acting over a longer period of time. Postures that increase force on the lower neck over a long period of time therefore apply significant pressure to the neck discs.

Third, the sensitivity of the pain pathways in the spinal cord and brain determine the amount of electricity produced in the brain. The longer the

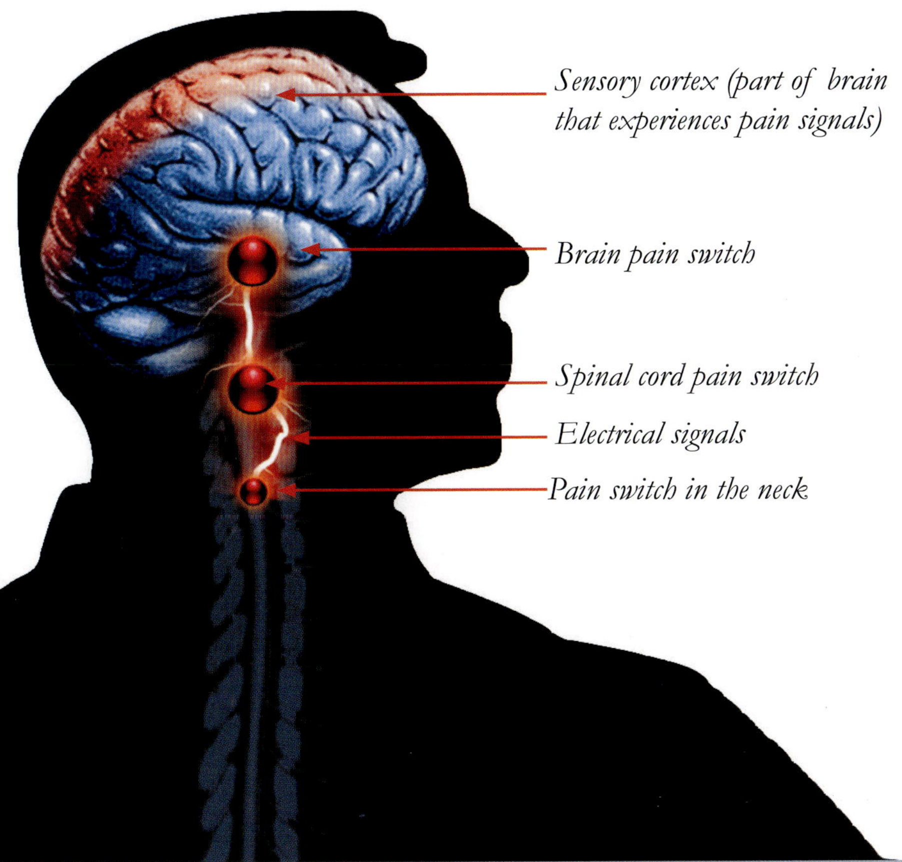

Figure 2.1
The pain pathways from the pain switch in the neck to the spinal cord and brain.

pain is present, the more sensitive the brain and spinal cord become to pain.

So what determines the sensitivity of your pain pathways? Your sensitivity to pain is often hereditary and can be increased by stress chemicals. Migraine is a condition that predisposes a person to amplify all sensations including pain, light, sound, smell and touch. Electrical channels are present in the brain that open more easily and spark increased amounts of electricity, resulting in heightened sensations. Therefore, during migraine attacks, harmless sensations such as light and sound become uncomfortable, and lying in a dark and quiet room is preferred.

For any given injury in the neck, a person who experiences migraine will experience more intense pain. Moreover, a migraine sufferer who is under stress will experience even more pain. The stress chemicals can in fact activate migraine, explaining why migraine sufferers will experience frequent episodes of migraine headache when under stress and then have minimal symptoms for several months.

Why does your pain become worse when you get stressed? The answer lies in the fact that stress chemicals can attach to your pain pathways and increase electricity, increasing the intensity of pain. Unfortunately, pain itself can cause the body to release stress chemicals. This can lead to a vicious cycle whereby pain creates stress chemicals that in turn amplify pain, leading to an ever-worsening experience of pain for the patient.

There are two other problems that can arise from the release of stress chemicals: the development of stress-related illnesses, such as insomnia, anxiety and depression; and the spread of pain to other parts of the body, known as referred pain. Once pain has spread there is no simple explanation for the cause of patients' symptoms. If pain is experienced only in the neck, doctors can easily deduce that a structure in the neck is likely to be the source. If pain spreads into the head, shoulder, arm or even throughout the body, diagnosing the problem is more difficult.

Another important question is what determines which activities will hurt and which activities will be pain-free. For neck pain, activities that increase pressure on damaged structures, such as the discs, will be painful. Looking down for long periods will increase pressure on the discs in the lower neck and often cause pain. Rotating the neck when backing the car may also cause pain. Sitting still for long periods of time at the computer is likely to increase pressure on the neck discs and can aggravate existing pain.

In summary, pain is experienced when a receptor detects an injury to a body part and creates an electrical spark that is transmitted to the brain to create the sensation of pain. Switches in the spinal cord and brain are capable of amplifying or diminishing pain. The amount of pain experienced depends on the extent of damage, pressure and the brain's pain sensitivity.

Referred pain

Referred pain is experienced at a site other than the original site of pain[2]. People who experience neck pain may also experience pain in the back of their shoulder, arms and head due to two separate reasons.

First, the brain may perceive the pain to be arising from the head, posterior shoulder or arm, when it is in fact arising from the neck. There is no damage to the head, posterior shoulder or arm even though pain is experienced at these sites.

As the intensity of pain increases, referred pain spreads further. As neck pain increases, pain may spread to the posterior shoulder, head and arms, as shown in Figure 2.2. However, once neck pain improves, the pain localises back into the neck.

When pain is localised to the neck, the electrical signal in the brain where pain

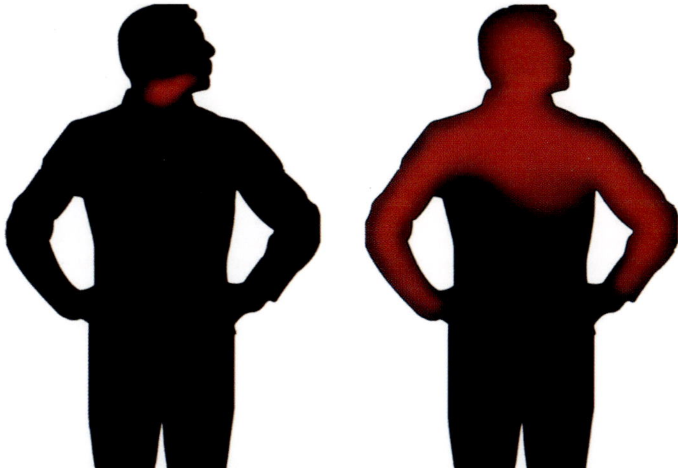

Figure 2.2

The image on the left shows mild pain from the neck that is restricted to the neck. The image on the right shows where pain can spread to with increasing severity of neck pain.

is represented is restricted to the neck as shown in Figure 2.3. The image on the right shows the pain spreading further down the arm (shown in red) as the electrical signal in the brain pain map spreads down the arm, causing the person to experience referred pain in the arm. The electrical impulses in the brain pain switch spread as the intensity and duration of pain increases. Figure 2.3 shows the electrical representation of neck pain in the brain pain map.

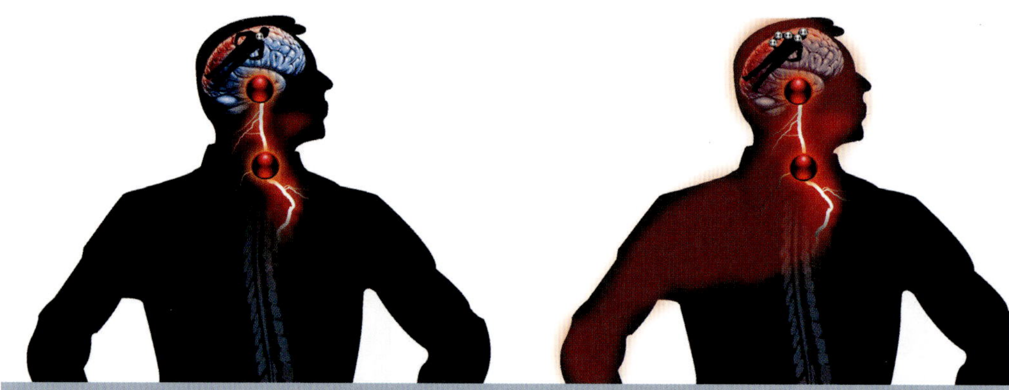

Figure 2.3

When pain is mild (left side picture), the pain arising from the neck is experienced only in the neck, with electrical signals confined to the neck region in the brain. The right hand picture shows how pain can spread from the neck into the head, shoulder and arm regions (shown in red) due to increase electrical signals in the brain pain map.

The second reason neck pain can spread symptoms into the arm and hand is because long nerves that start in the neck extend to those areas. These nerves can be irritated in the neck when they are compressed by a prolapsed disc (Figure 2.4), resulting in symptoms of sharp shooting pain, pins and needles, numbness and tingling in the arm and hand. Weakness can also develop as the nerves are instrumental in maintaining power to the muscles of the arm and hand. Symptoms from nerve irritation are often experienced in one arm but can be experienced in both, depending on the size and spread of the disc prolapse.

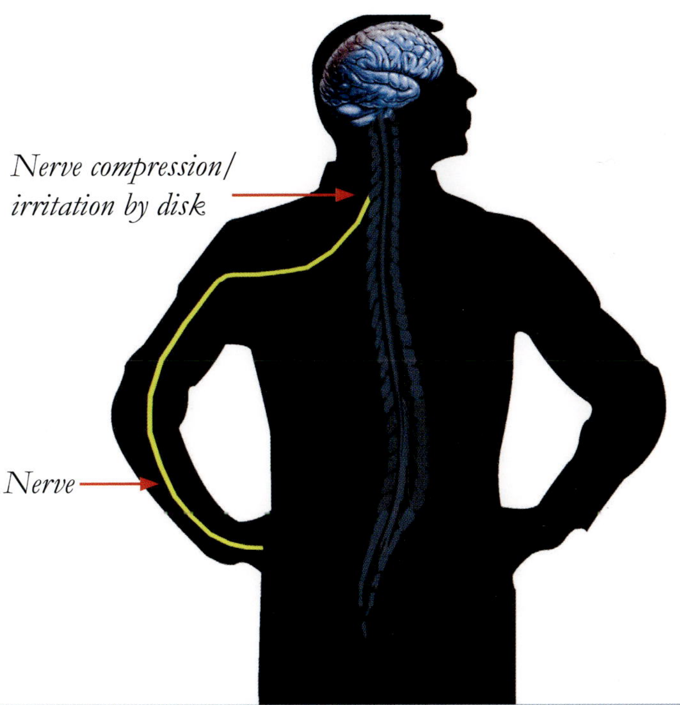

Figure 2.4

The nerves that exit in the neck travel down the arm and hand. When they are compressed or irritated as they exit the neck they can cause pain, pins and needles, numbness and tingling down the arm as far as the fingers.

Nerve compression and referred pain spread pain beyond the soure of the patients' symptoms. Knowing what is the source of the pain is essential to managing and alleviating pain. Chapter 3 examines the various sources of neck pain.

CASE STUDY: *Catherine*

Catherine came to my clinic in February 2014 after a motor vehicle accident in April 2012, experiencing significant neck pain. She was on the motorway and hit the car in front of her before she was then rear-ended by the car behind her. Her neck pain continued after the accident and had increased over the following year.

Catherine worked as a beauty therapist, requiring her to look down for long periods of time. This was aggravating her symptoms, which had spread from her neck to her shoulders and down the arms. She had pins and needles in her fingers and had also noticed her whole left arm sometimes had a very light tingling sensation. To her surprise, she was also experiencing symptoms in both feet. She sometimes felt like she was walking on glass. She also started experiencing frequent headaches. A few months prior to her consultation she had to stop work.

An MRI scan (Figure 2.5) showed there was a disc prolapse (commonly called a slipped disc) and there was compression of the layer surrounding the spinal cord. Most of Catherine's symptoms were due to referred pain from her disc. The looking down required in her work increased the pressure on the disc further, causing the disc to squeeze onto the nerve, creating pins and needles down the arm and hand. The pressure also increased the severity of her neck pain.

Catherine started using a traction collar, stretching her neck, and wore a soft collar when performing activities in which she needed to look down. Within a week she noted that the symptoms in her feet, as well as the light tingling sensation in her left arm were gone. Her pain reduced mostly to the posterior neck.

Catherine has returned to work in modified activities with many of her symptoms improved.

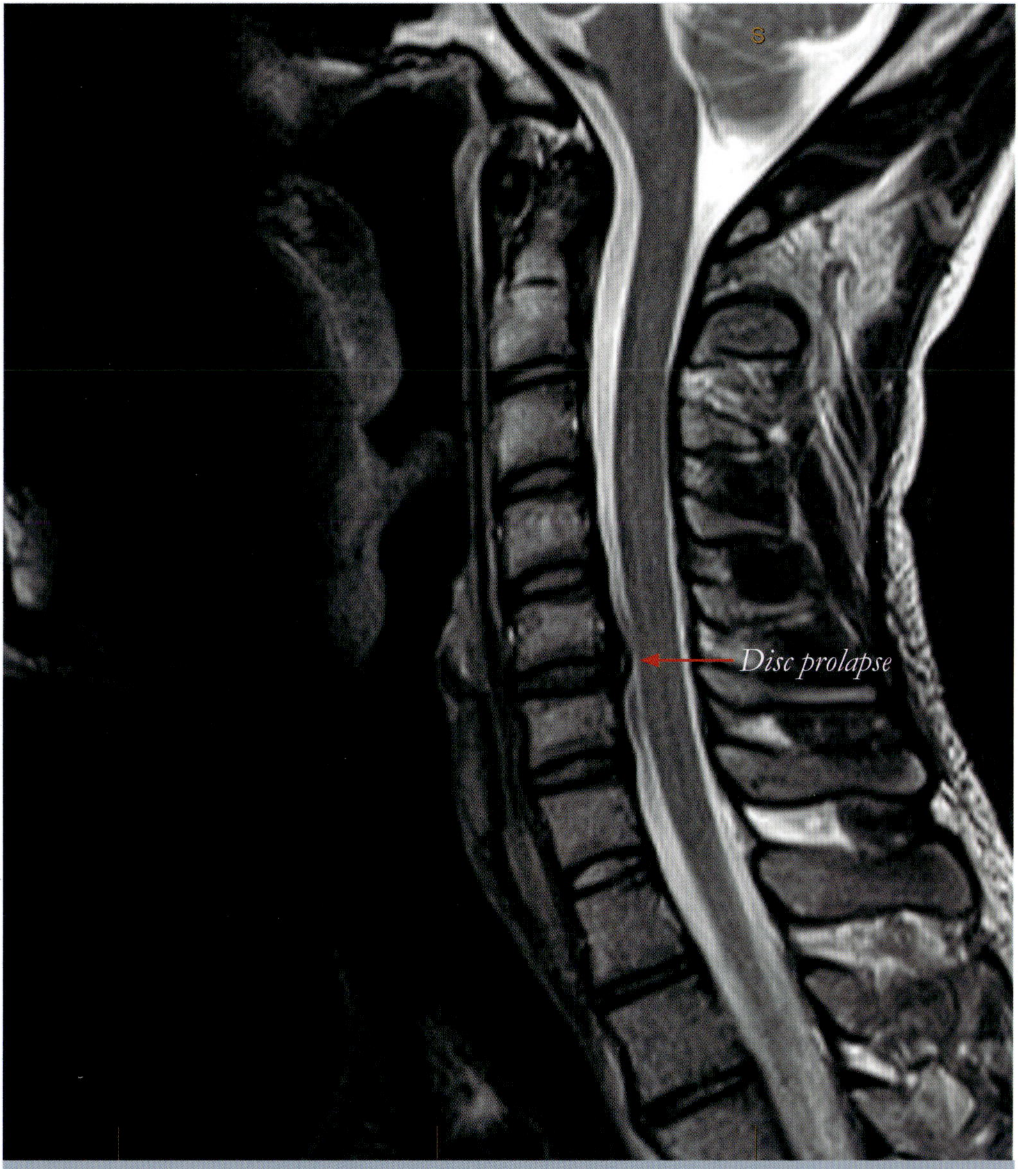

Figure 2.5
A disc prolapse is seen between the fifth and sixth vertebrae in the neck.

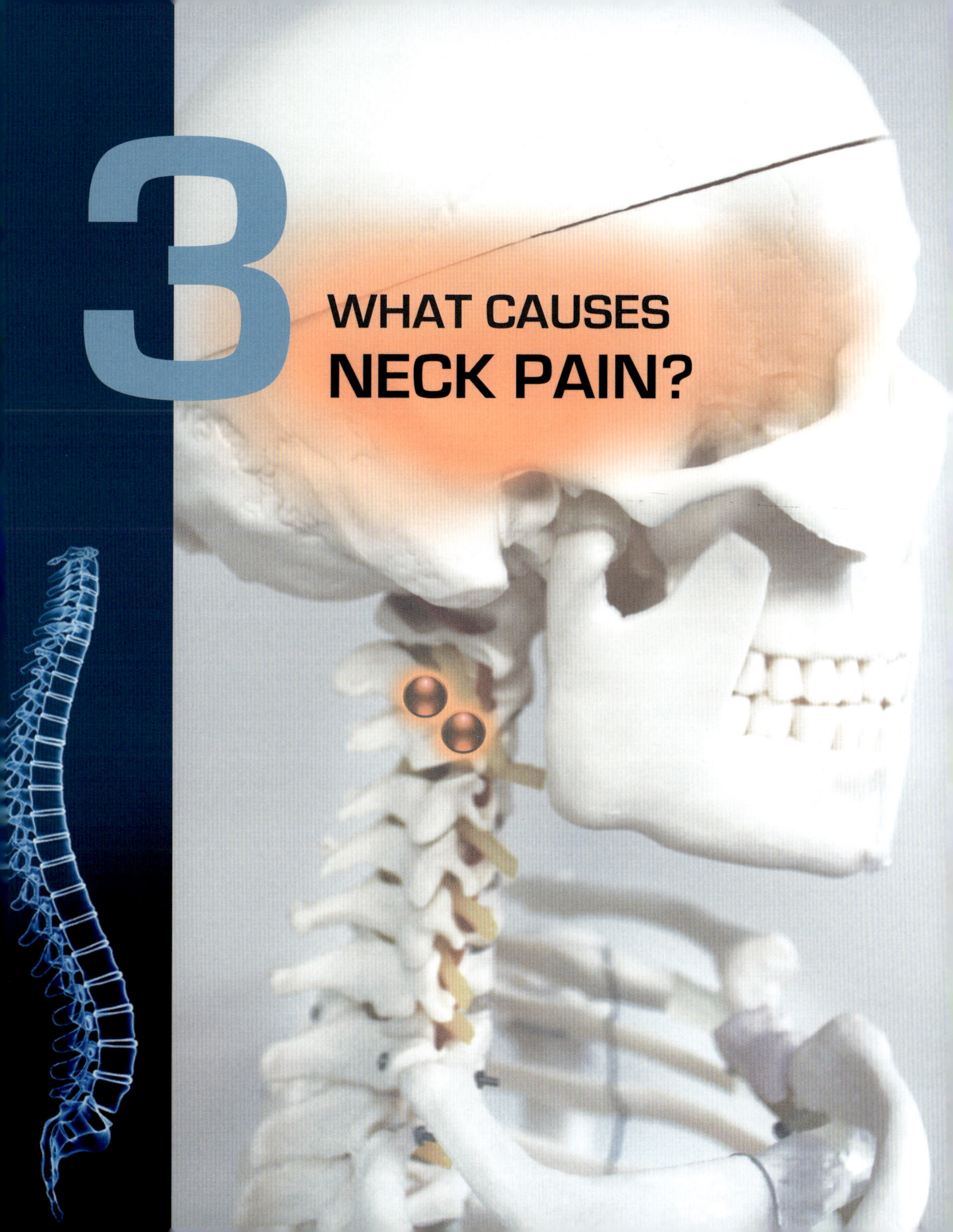

3 WHAT CAUSES NECK PAIN?

The spinal column consists of 24 bones called vertebrae, with discs in between that act as shock absorbers and allow flexibility of the spine. At the top of the spinal column, the neck consists of seven vertebrae labelled C1 to C7 – as previously stated, the medical term for the neck. Contained within these vertebrae is the spinal cord, a collection of nerves from the brain that communicate with the whole body.

The discs become more prominent at the lower levels of the neck as they are required to absorb increased forces. Pairs of joints at the back of the spine, called the facet joints, prevent excessive movement of the neck. There are also several ligaments in front of and behind the neck that help stabilise the neck.

As previously stated, any structure with a nerve supply in the neck is capable of causing pain, including the bones, joints, disc, ligaments, muscles and tendons. Sometimes, pain may also be referred to the shoulder, arm and head from any structure in the neck.

Whenever a deeper structure causes pain, the electrical signals spread into all the muscles of the neck, head, shoulders and even arms. Muscle knots develop which can become another source of pain. Once muscle tightness occurs, joint tightness can also develop within the neck. A person may damage a disc in the neck and then develop muscle spasm and joint tightness in the months following the injury. Once this happens, the disc, muscle and joints need to be treated, otherwise full resolution may not occur.

Whiplash is the term given to the movement of the neck during trauma such as falls or car accidents. It is essentially a quick motion when the neck moves forwards and then backwards (or backwards and then forwards) as shown in Figure 3.2. Although commonly associated with motor vehicle accidents, whiplash-type injuries can occur with any fall or impact injury. Whiplash events can injure several of the structures in the neck, including muscles, ligaments, joints and discs. The head acts as a significant weight in a whiplash injury and increases the chance of injuring a neck structure.

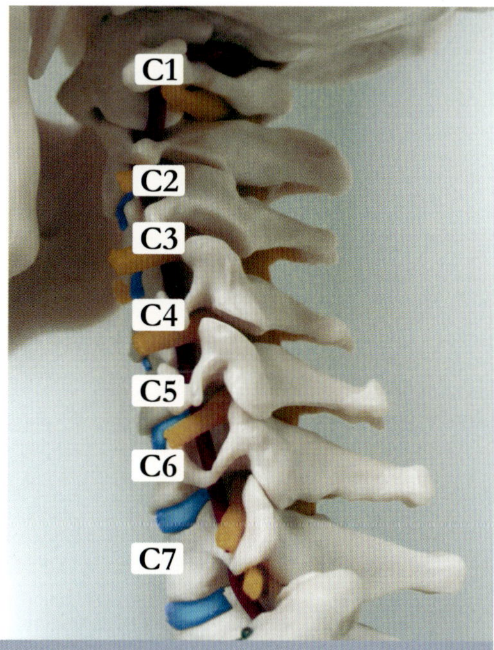

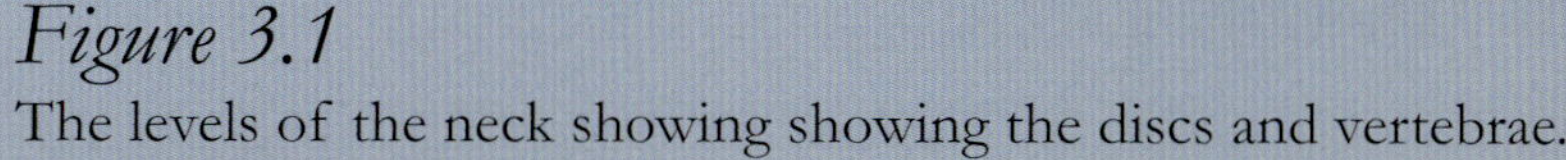

Figure 3.1
The levels of the neck showing showing the discs and vertebrae.

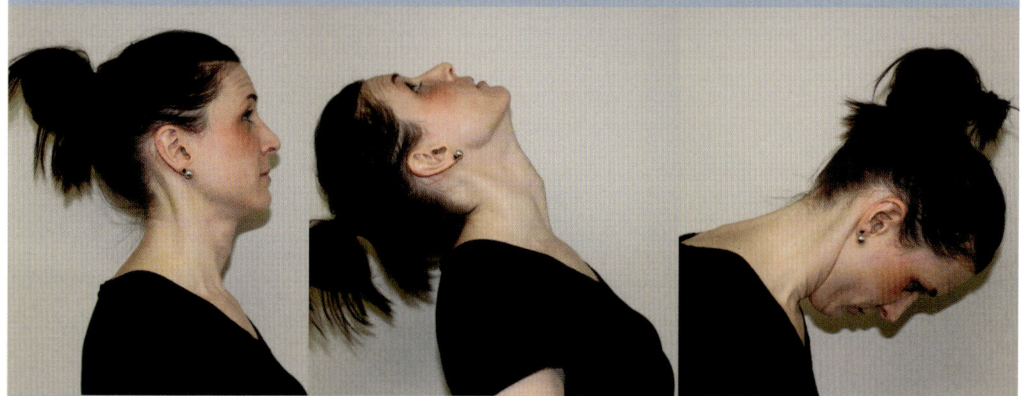

Figure 3.2
The sequence of events in a whiplash-type injury includes extension followed by flexion of the neck.

The muscles of the neck

The muscles surrounding the neck can cause pain and refer pain into the head, shoulder and arm regions. The referral pattern of neck muscles has been extensively researched, and a sample of these is shown in Figures 3.4 to 3.8.

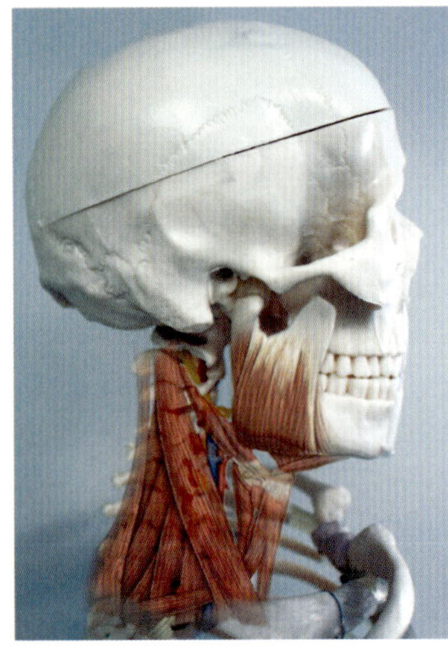

Figure 3.3
There are several groups of muscles that surround the neck.

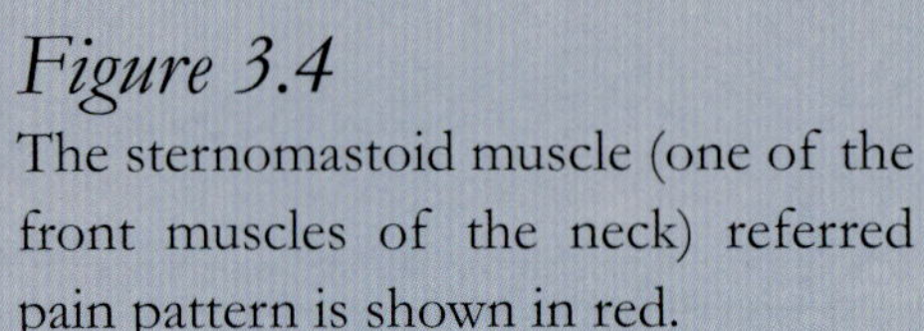

Figure 3.4
The sternomastoid muscle (one of the front muscles of the neck) referred pain pattern is shown in red.

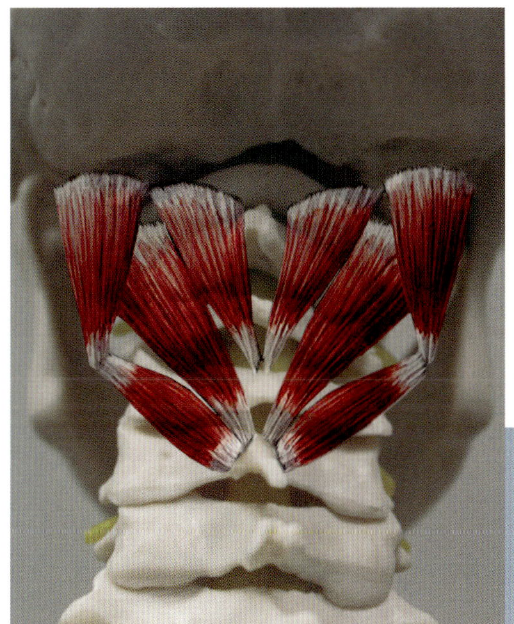

Figure 3.5
The suboccipital muscles are shown at the back of the head and neck.

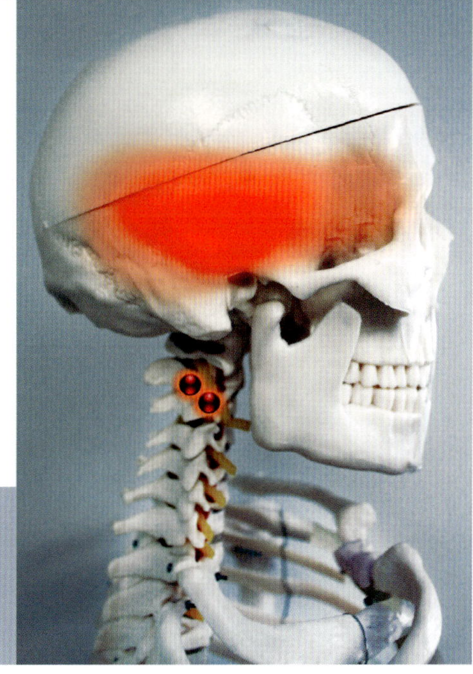

Figure 3.6
The suboccipital muscles refer pain into the side of the head and behind the eye.

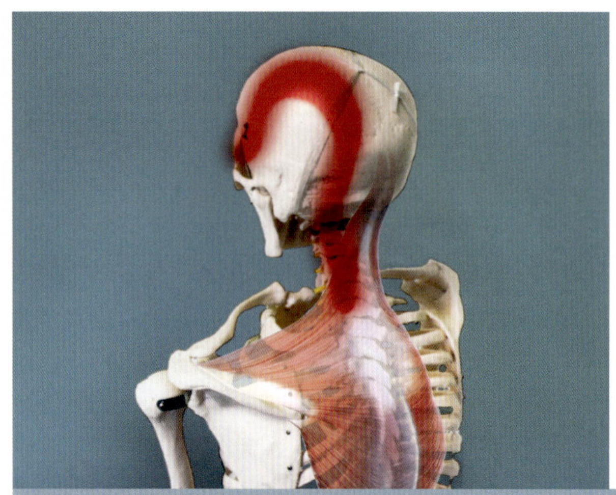

Figure 3.7
The pattern of pain arising from one of the largest muscles of the neck (trapezius).

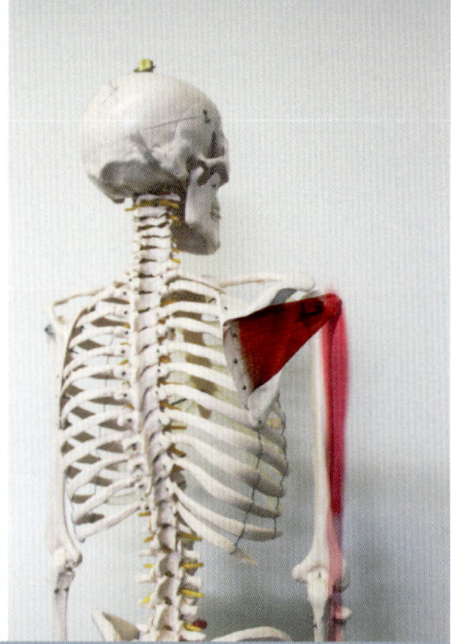

Figure 3.8
The pattern of pain arising from a posterior shoulder muscle (infraspinatus muscle).

The ligaments and tendons

Ligaments are leather-strap-like structures that hold two bones together, while tendons attach a muscle to bone. There are several tendons and ligaments surrounding the neck that can cause pain around the head and neck region. There is no definite test to diagnose ligament pain, but examination may reveal tenderness. Some ligaments can become torn in high-impact injuries and cause instability of the bones, allowing them more movement than normal. Intact ligaments, in contrast, often usefully restrict movement between bones. If treatment aimed at tendons or ligaments successfully reduces pain, it can be assumed these structures were contributing to pain. Treatment of ligaments and tendons may include manual therapies such as friction massage, electrical therapies or injections. Injection solutions include steroids, anaesthetic, prolotherapy or saline.

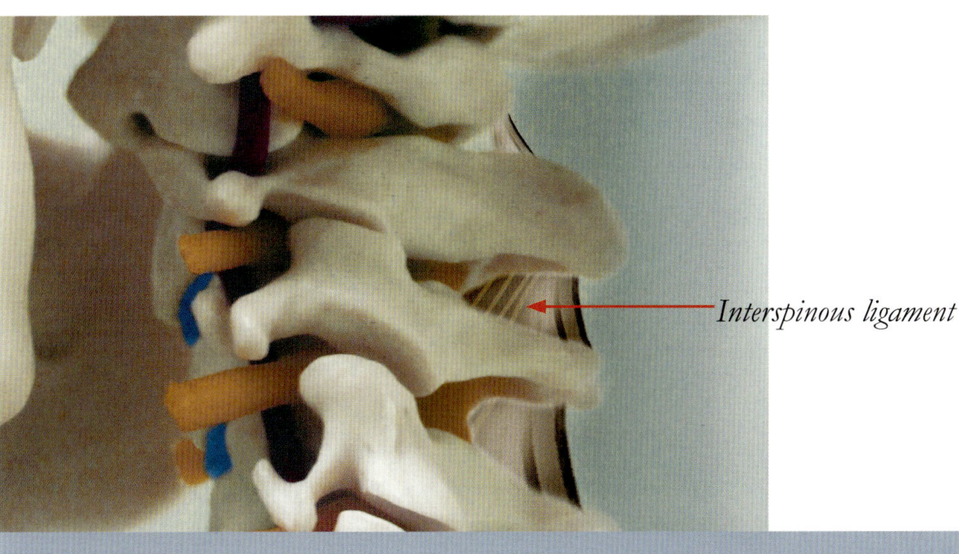

Figure 3.9
The ligaments at the back of the neck (interspinous ligaments) are shown.

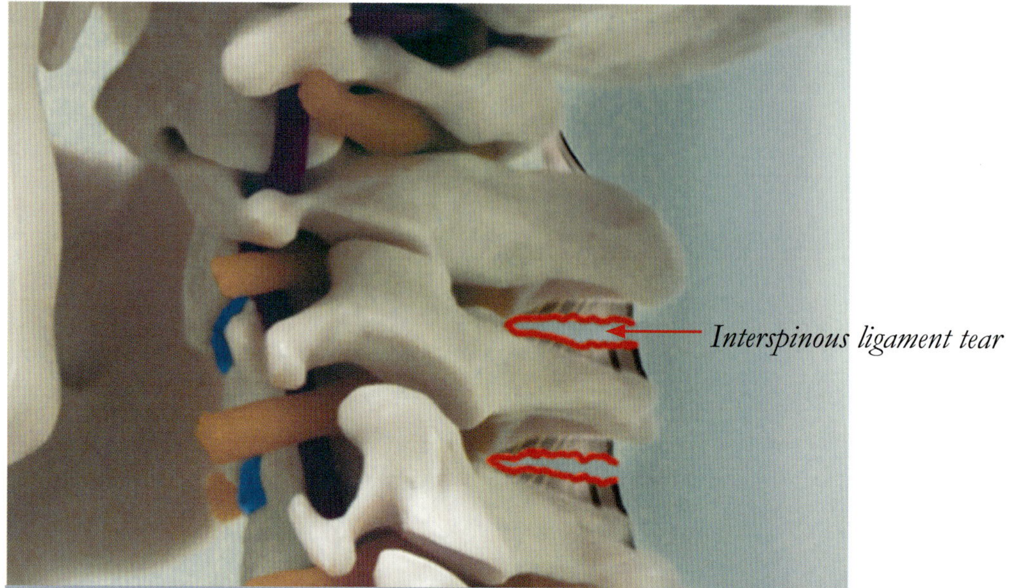

Figure 3.10
Ligaments of the cervical spine can be torn due to major trauma such as whiplash injury.

The disc

The disc is a unique structure that acts as a shock absorber and allows flexibility of the spine. If the spine were a single long bone, it would crack easily as the body moves. The disc is sandwiched between two vertebrae (bones) as shown in Figure 3.11. The discs become more prominent in the lower neck as the forces absorbed by the discs increase.

The outside wall of the disc is the annular ligament (ring ligament) and the centre of the disc is made up of gel (Figure 3.12). The gel can consist of up to 90% water. The ring ligament is composed of thin fibrous layers that are fused together. The layers are actually criss-crossed to give the ring ligament

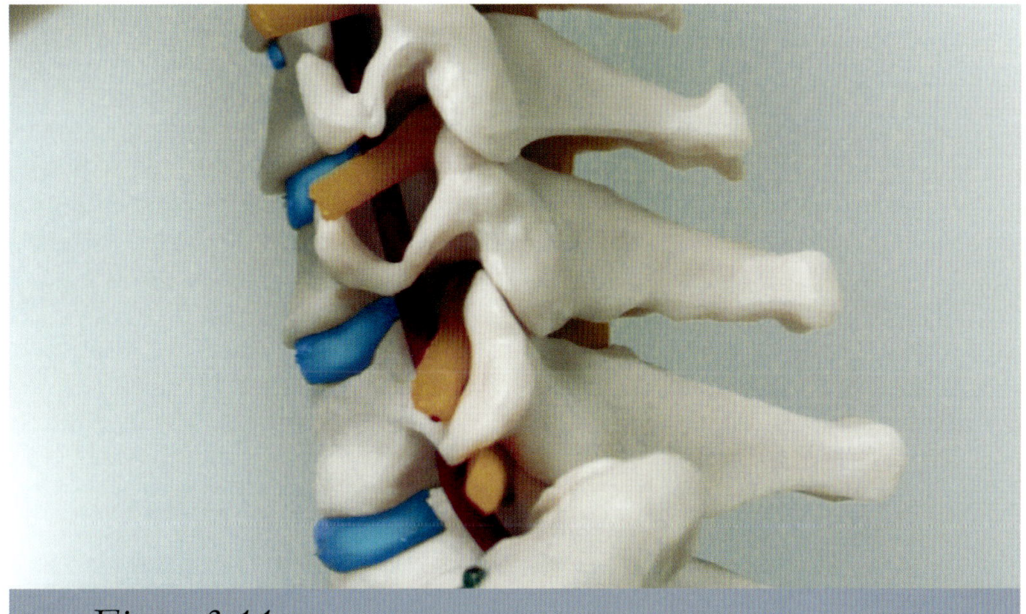

Figure 3.11
The discs (shown in blue) are arranged between the bones. They are are designed to absorb pressure and allow flexibility of the spine.

incredible strength. The top and bottom of the disc are covered by a thin plate called the endplate that allows diffusion of nutrients and water into and out of the disc.

Very large forces are often transmitted onto the disc when a person performs activities when looking down. The pressure placed on the discs in the lower neck can increase by 10 times in this position. The ring ligament and gel centre have been found to absorb half the pressure each. The disc acts like a hydraulic system as shown in Figure 3.13. When pressure is exerted on the gel, it is distributed evenly throughout the ring ligament, regardless of which way the spine bends. Although the ring ligament is very strong, it can develop tears due to accidents such as falls or motor vehicle injuries. It may even deteriorate due to poor posture. The layers of the ring ligament can separate and some of the inner layers of the ring can tear from repeated pressure.

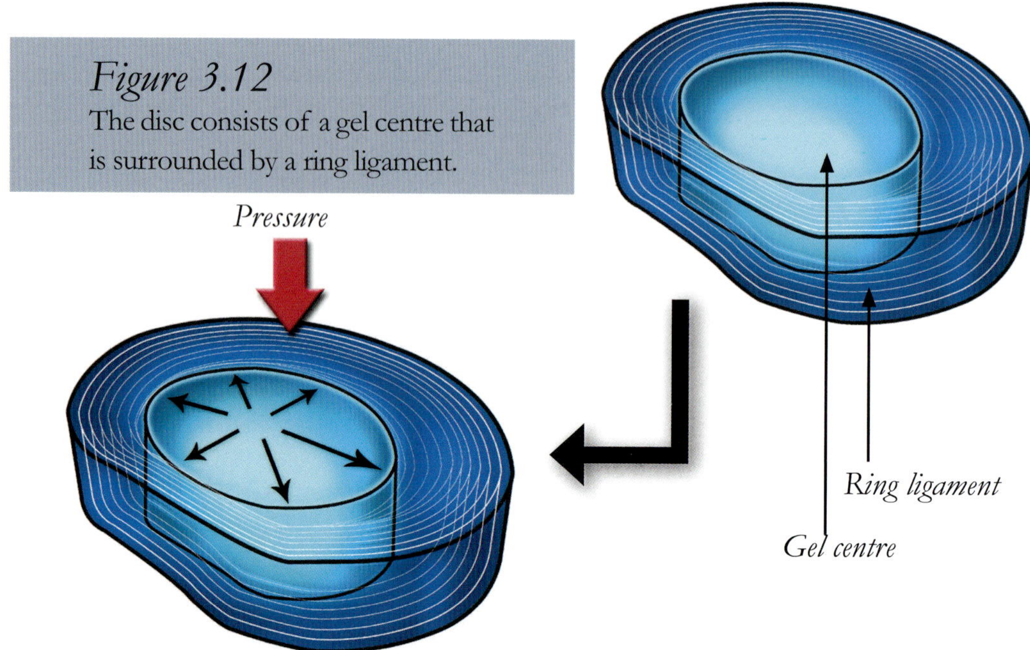

Figure 3.12
The disc consists of a gel centre that is surrounded by a ring ligament.

Figure 3.13
The disc acts like a hydraulic piece of machinery with the gel in the middle of the ring ligament spreading pressure to all parts of the disc wall.

The ring ligament can therefore become filled with the gel oozing from the centre of the disc, as shown in Figure 3.14. Once the disc is damaged, the gel loses its water gradually over time. In its healthy state, the gel is composed of fine filaments that attract water. But once the gel enters the ring, enzymes are activated that break down the fine filaments. When the fine filaments break down, the gel no longer holds water and becomes dehydrated. So what happens to the hydraulic function of the disc once the gel becomes dry? The pressure within the gel no longer spreads evenly around the ligament. Instead, the torn portion of the ring ligament is stretched, creating a disc bulge as shown in Figure 3.15. A bulge can progress to the point that the entire width of the ligament develops a tear. A disc prolapse occurs when the gel protrudes out of the ring ligament as shown in Figure 3.16.

Figure 3.14
A torn ring ligament filled with the gel.

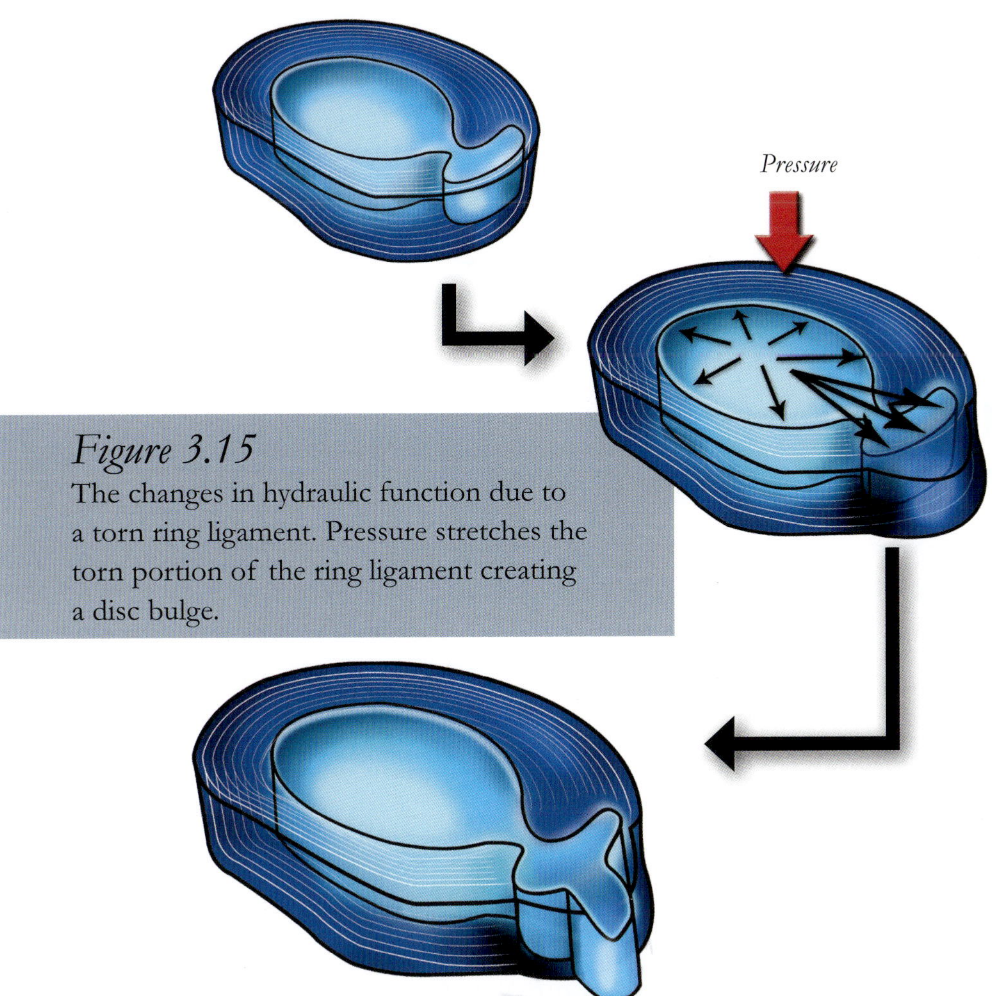

Figure 3.15
The changes in hydraulic function due to a torn ring ligament. Pressure stretches the torn portion of the ring ligament creating a disc bulge.

Figure 3.16
In a disc prolapse the gel protrudes out of the ring ligament.

A disc prolapse can cause pressure on the nerve that exits near the disc, as shown in Figure 3.17. The nerves that exit the neck are long and can extend as far as the fingers. Irritation or pressure on these nerves can result in sharp, shooting, severe pain that extends to the fingers as shown in Figure 3.18. Pins and needles and tingling can also extend to the fingers. These nerves control muscle power and the sensation in the skin of the arm and hand. Disruption of this nerve signal may cause both weakness and numbness.

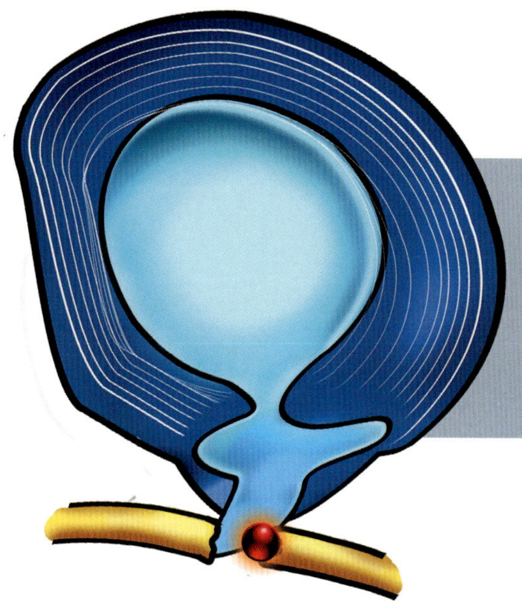

Figure 3.17
The centre gel can squeeze through the wall of the disc (disc prolapse) and irritate the nerve that travels down the arm.

The pain suffered by those with a slipped disc pressing on a nerve is severe and would be like striking your funny bone and then keeping the funny bone pressed against a table for days, weeks or even months. If pressure continues on the nerve for long periods of time, numbness and weakness in the arm may become permanent. Fortunately a slipped disc will usually shrink in time, with nerve symptoms reducing accordingly.

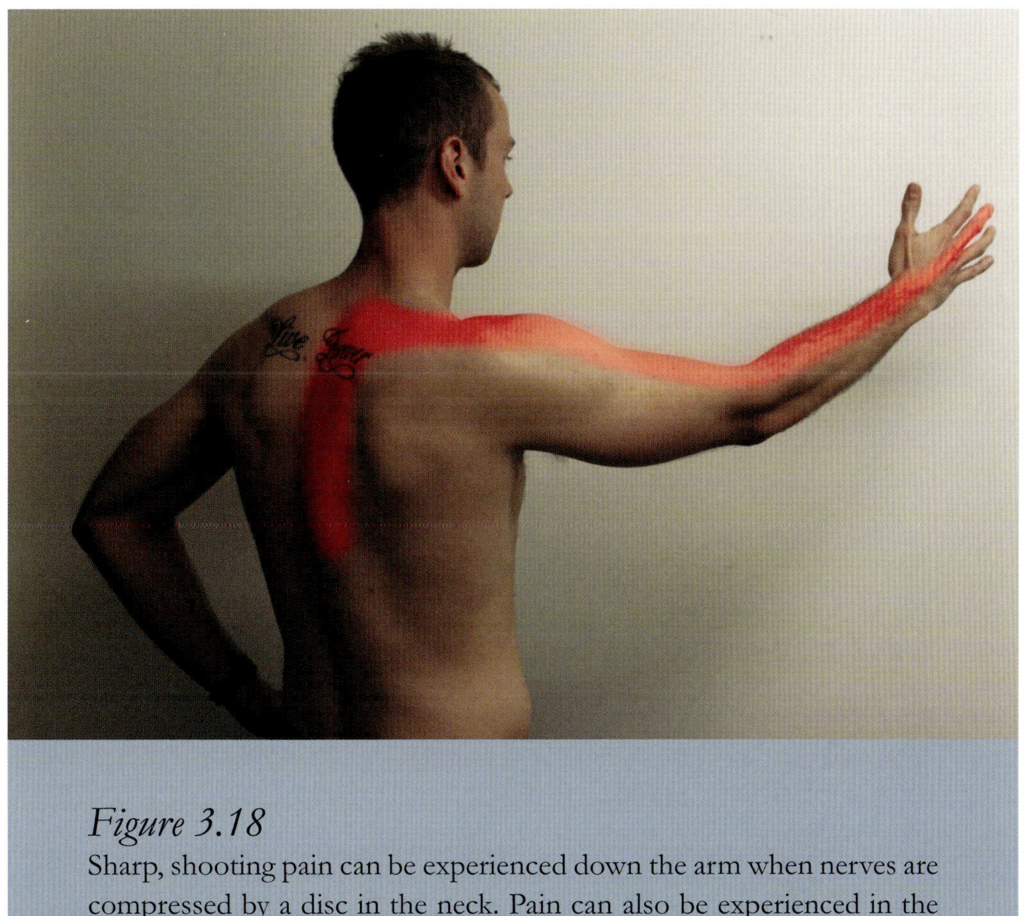

Figure 3.18
Sharp, shooting pain can be experienced down the arm when nerves are compressed by a disc in the neck. Pain can also be experienced in the posterior shoulder.

When you looks down, the weight of your head doubles for every 10 degrees of flexion. So an average 5kg head when upright exerts 45kg of pressure on the lower neck when you are is looking down 90 degrees. This pressure causes electrical signals to form in the disc and adjacent bony surfaces that can be experienced as pain. Furthermore the increased pressure on the discs causes them to squeeze outwards, which can irritate the nerves that supply the arms.

Discs can cause pain due to pressure mostly from the weight of the head. The patterns of disc pain from different levels can vary[3] as shown in Figure 3.19.

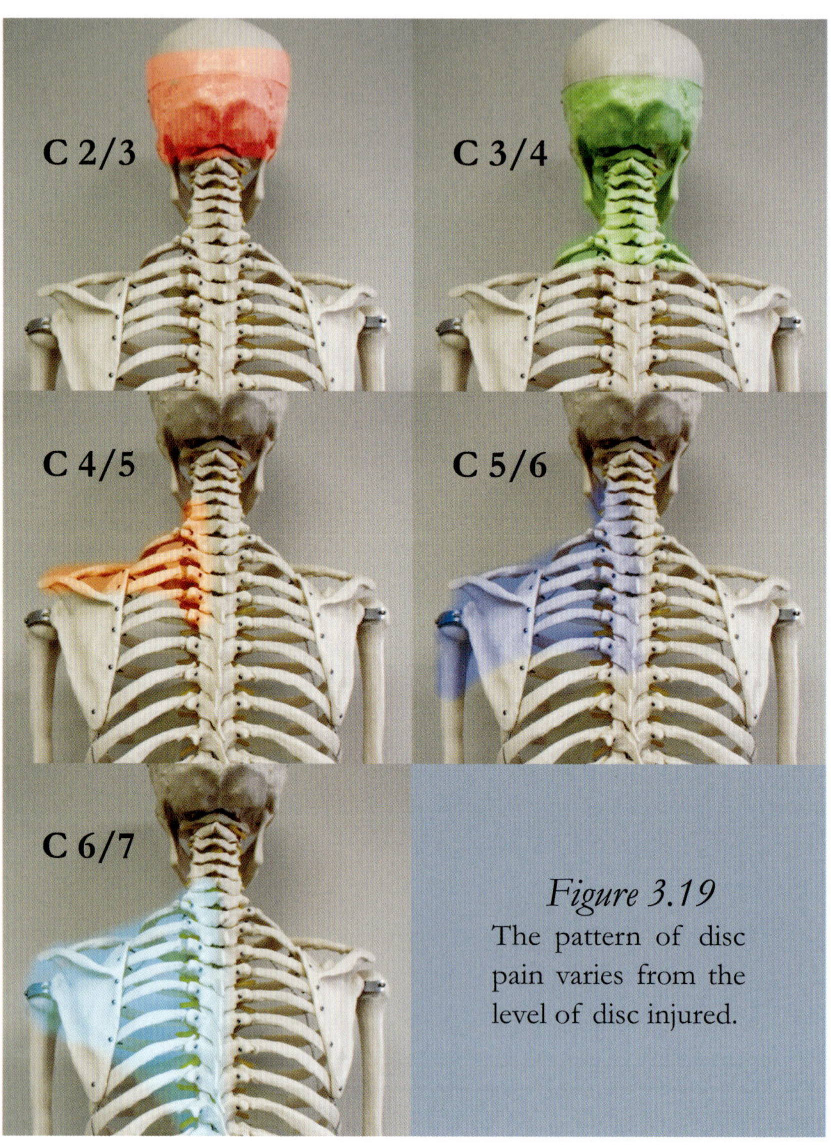

Figure 3.19
The pattern of disc pain varies from the level of disc injured.

CASE STUDY: *Sue*

In 2009 Sue was trying to get fit, and while performing sit-ups developed pain in the neck. Over the next week she also developed tingling in the left hand. The pain increased despite therapy, and she was taking analgesics and tablets to help her sleep. She found that working at her laptop and computer aggravated her symptoms the most.

Despite experiencing symptoms for a year before seeing me, she did not know what was causing them. An MRI scan (Figure 3.20) showed a disc prolapse that was causing her neck pain as well as compressing a nerve that supplies the left hand.

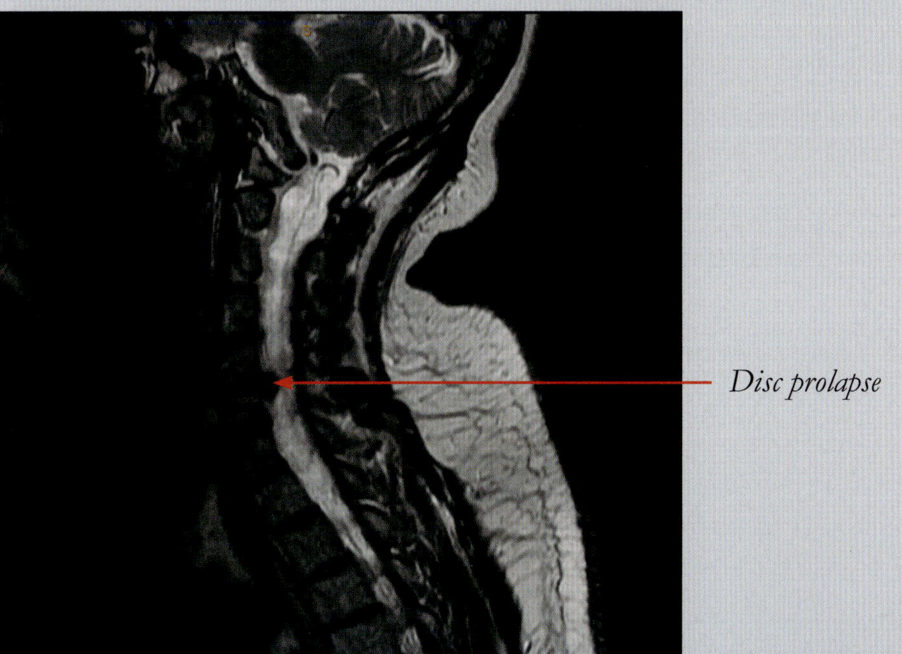

Figure 3.20
An MRI scan shows a disc prolapse between the fifth and sixth vertebrae. The disc is also narrowed.

The head puts considerable pressure on the neck discs due to gravity. When there is no loading of the disc, for instance in a lying down posture, the water returns to the gel from the bone, as shown in Figure 3.21. When sitting upright for long periods, such as when working at a computer, the fluid within the disc diffuses into the adjacent vertebrae as shown in Figure 3.22. The disc becomes harder and less able to absorb pressure, subsequently placing more pressure on the bones. This reduces the height of the disc, as shown in Figure 3.23. Often a person will injure their disc and then experience repeated episodes of neck pain whenever they irritate the injured disc. Long-term changes can occur to the disc once it is damaged. When the gel loses water, it no longer absorbs its half share of the pressure, meaning the ring ligament absorbs most of the pressure and becomes squashed over years and decades, as shown in Figure 3.24. After many years the disc starts to reduce in height.

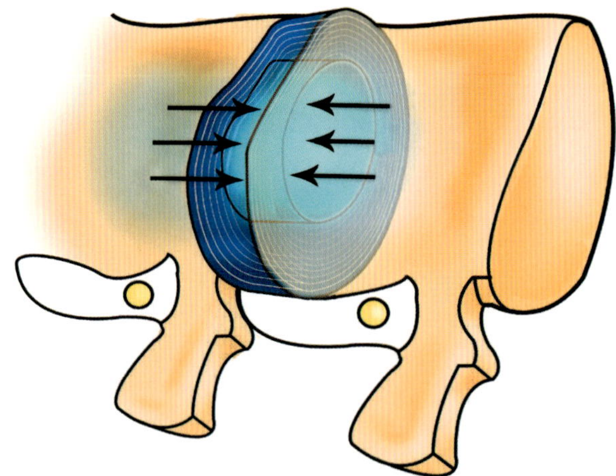

Figure 3.21

When lying down, gravity is removed and the water returns from the adjacent bones into the gel of the disc. Disc height is regained.

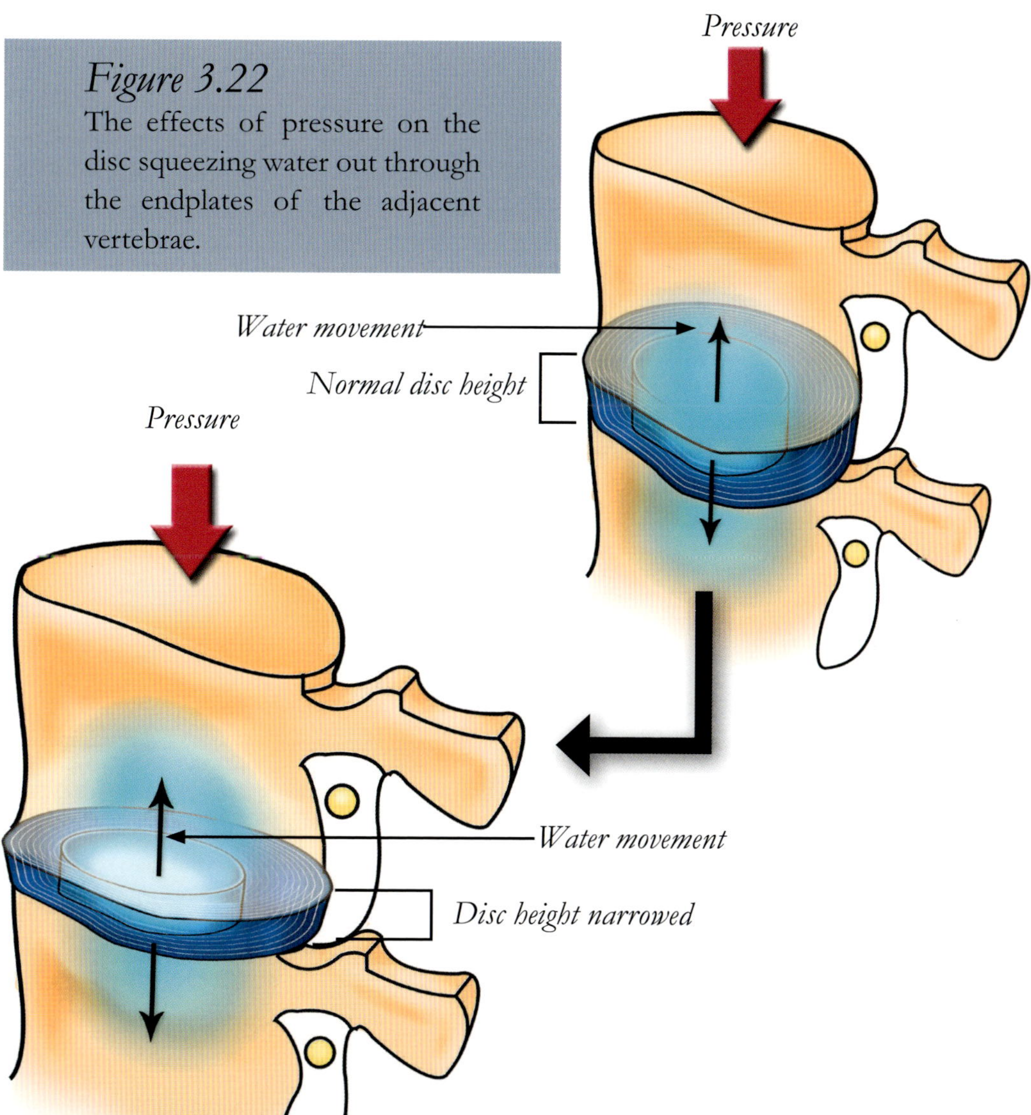

Figure 3.22
The effects of pressure on the disc squeezing water out through the endplates of the adjacent vertebrae.

Figure 3.23
The disc narrows in the upright posture over the course of the day. Activities that load the neck such as flexion of the head can increase the narrowing that occurs due to increased pressure on the disc.

The reduction in disc height can take many years or decades and can be seen on an X-ray after many years as a narrowed gap between two vertebrae. As the disc decomes dehydrated and narrowed, increased pressure falls on the vertebrae creating bony spurs (osteophytes). The combination of narrowed discs and bony spurs is often termed degenerative change on radiology reports. Sometimes these changes are referred to as arthritis of the spine.

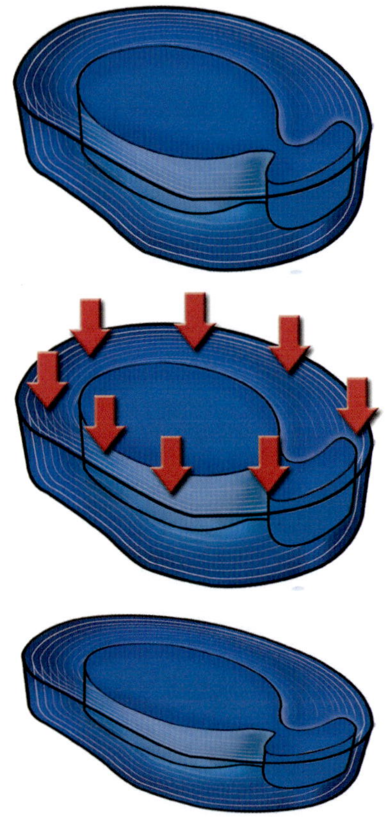

Figure 3.24

The gel dries out and increased pressure falls on the ring ligament. After years the ligament becomes squashed and loses height.

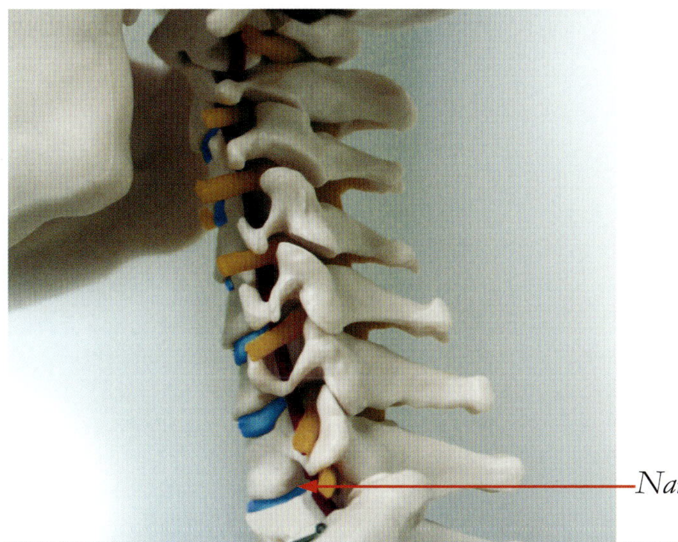

Figure 3.25
Once a disc has been damaged, over several years it can narrow and become less able to absorb pressure.

As time passes, significant changes occur in the bony ends of the vertebrae adjacent to an injured disc. Extra nerves and blood vessels form in response to the extra pressure that falls on the end of the vertebrae. The end becomes more sensitive as a result of the nerves as they detect pressure and create electrical sparks, which in turn is experienced as pain. Compounding the problem are the previously described changes in the disc, such as the loss of water in the gel that changes the disc from a fluid structure to a more solid structure. This in turn puts more pressure on the vertebrae. The combination of increased sensitivity of the bony surfaces and a more solid disc increases the likelihood of pain from these structures. Fortunately, once a person adopts better postures that reduce pressure on the disc, or makes use of treatments such as collars and traction therapy (as described in Chapter 5), the increased nerves are likely to wither away, leaving the bones less sensitive to pressure and leading to a reduction in pain.

Facet joints

The small joints that sit behind the spine are called facet joints, as seen in Figure 3.26. Facet joints can be a source of neck pain. If the disc narrows, the joints come closer together and may press against each other, leading to pain. Pain arising from a facet joint in the neck can also radiate down into the posterior shoulder region, as shown in Figure 3.27. Pain arising from a facet joint in the neck can cause pain to radiate into the head as well as down the back of the shoulder blade, as shown in Figure 3.27.

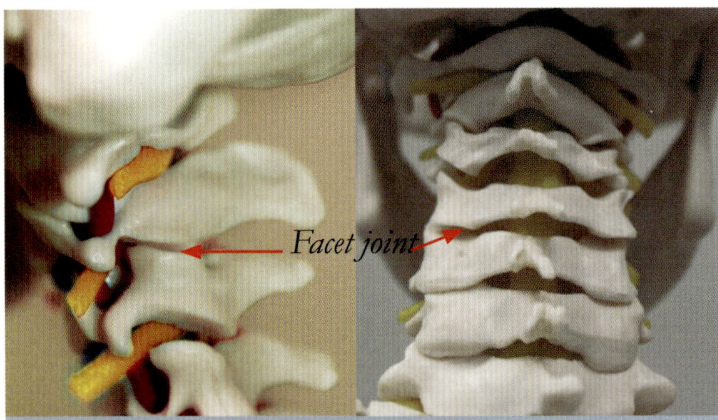

Figure 3.26

The left picture shows the facet joints in the neck from one side, while the right image shows the pairs of facet joints from behind.

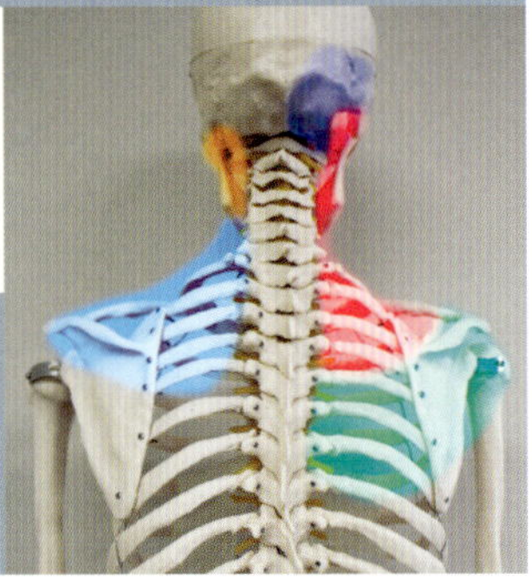

Figure 3.27

The area of referred pain from each facet joint is represented as a different colour.

The shoulder

Shoulder pain is often confused with neck pain and vice versa. The nerves that supply the neck also supply the shoulder muscles, resulting in similar patterns of pain from both, often causing confusion as to where the pain arises. Shoulder muscles can spread pain down the arm and into the neck (Figure 3.28) contributing to the confusion.

When people experience pain in the shoulder, neck and arm, the origin of the pain may be the neck, the shoulder or both the neck and shoulder. Sometimes trauma can damage both the neck and the shoulder and people can experience pain arising from both structures. If a person has a limited range of motion of the neck, pain on looking behind when backing a car, or pain when looking down for long periods, the neck may be a more likely source of symptoms. If a person can't move their shoulder fully, and in particular struggles to raise their arms above shoulder height, the shoulder is likely to be the source of pain.

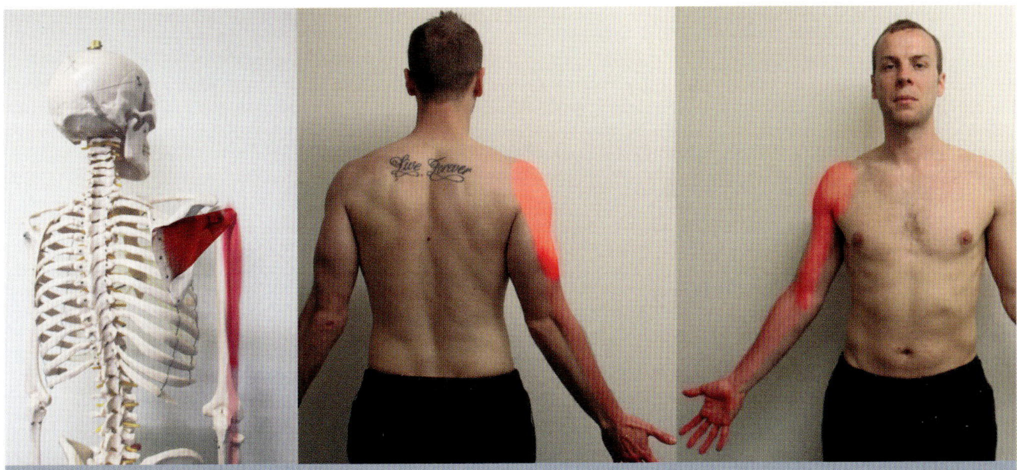

Figure 3.28 Shoulder muscles can refer pain well beyond the shoulder into the neck and down the arm.

CASE STUDY: *Paul*

Paul was water skiing one day, and, while getting up with his arms outstretched in front of him, experienced pain in the shoulder and neck region. Over many years he was treated for neck pain. A MRI scan of his neck (Figure 3.29) in 2012 confirmed disc damage and subsequent narrowing, most severely between the fifth and sixth vertebrae. Despite treatment of the neck, Paul also experienced pain in the left shoulder and had trouble sleeping on that shoulder. An ultrasound scan showed all four tendons were ruptured in the left shoulder. An X-ray of the left shoulder (Figure 3.30) showed arthritis. During the water skiing accident Paul had injured his left shoulder, but due to confusion the shoulder had never been investigated or treated, leading to arthritis developing. Paul went on to have a left shoulder replacement (Figure 3.31) that reduced his shoulder pain and enabled him to sleep better at night.

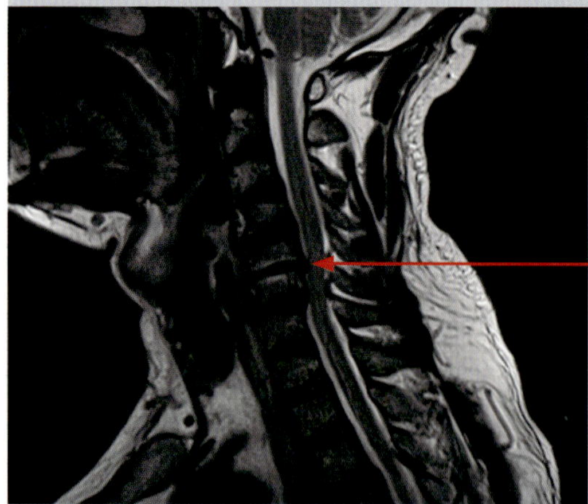

Figure 3.29
The MRI scan of the neck shows marked narrowing between the fifth and sixth neck vertebrae as well as lesser narrowing at the level below.

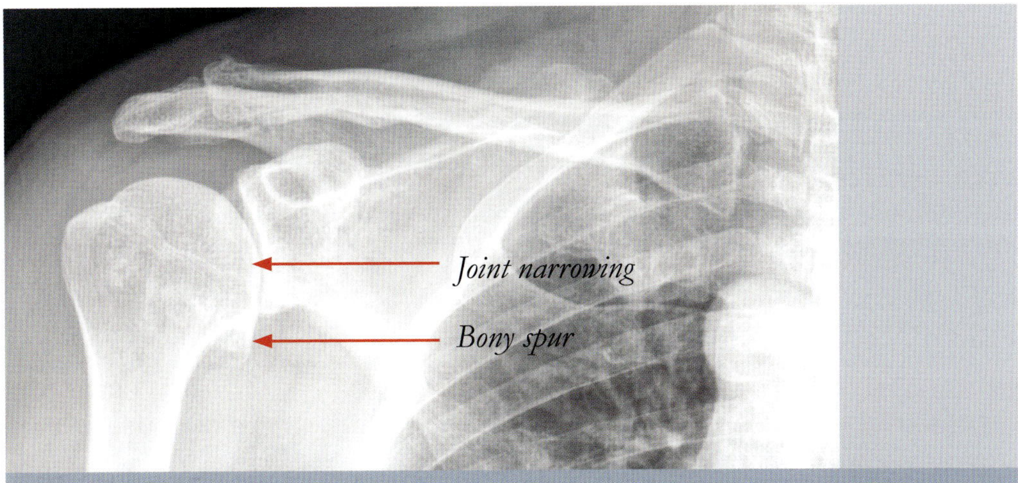

Figure 3.30
The shoulder X-ray shows the ball and socket of the shoulder have a minimal gap between them (arthritis) and that there is also a large bony spur at the lower end of the ball of the shoulder.

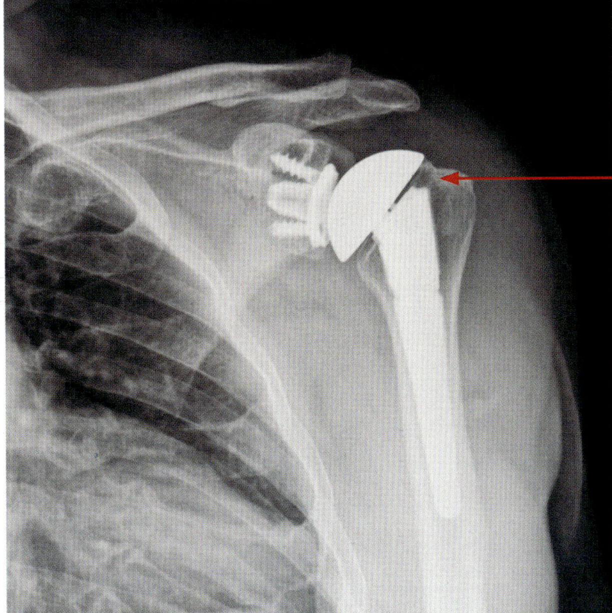

Figure 3.31
The shoulder joint has been replaced with an artificial joint.

Neck pain can cause changes in the shoulder that can in turn cause secondary shoulder problems. Neck pain can spread pain to all of the shoulder muscles, causing muscle contraction and altering the lengths and movement patterns of the muscles. When you raisie your arm above head height to comb your hair, reach up for high cupboards or hang washing on the line, the shoulder blade at the back of the shoulder must rotate, as shown in Figure 3.32.

If rotation is hampered by knots in the shoulder muscles, a structure called a bursa (named the subacromial bursa in the shoulder) becomes pinched under the tip of the collar bone as shown in Figure 3.33. An exaggerated curve in the mid back, as shown in Figure 3.34, can also reduce rotation of the shoulder blade. If this structure is repeatedly pinched, there is often pain when raising your arm above shoulder height and also when lying on your side while sleeping. Shoulder pain management must address any symptoms coming from your neck if it is to successfully reduce shoulder symptoms in the long term.

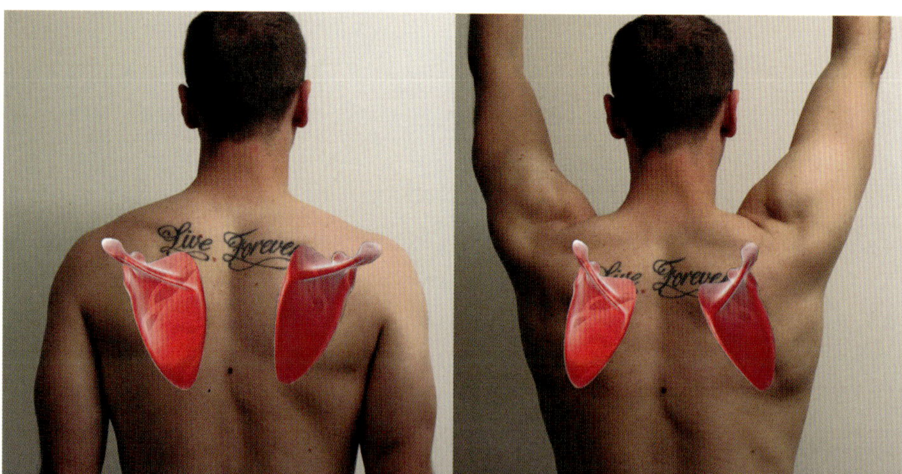

Figure 3.32

The scapula rotates outwards as shown when raising the shoulder. If the scapula does not rotate then the bursa become compressed and can cause pain.

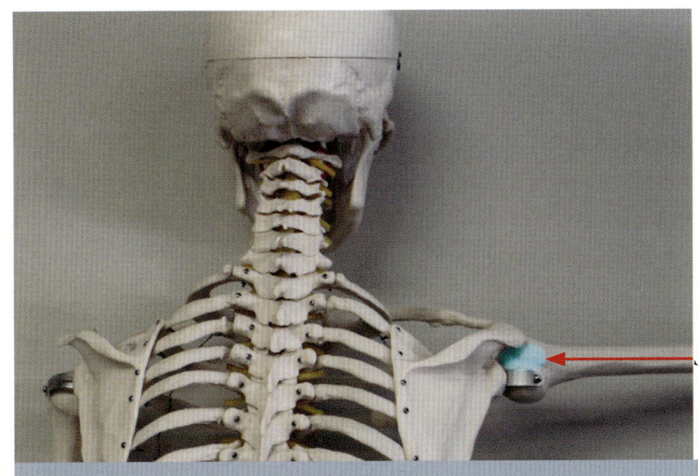

Figure 3.33
The bursa, shown in colour, becomes compressed when the arm is elevated and can result in pain.

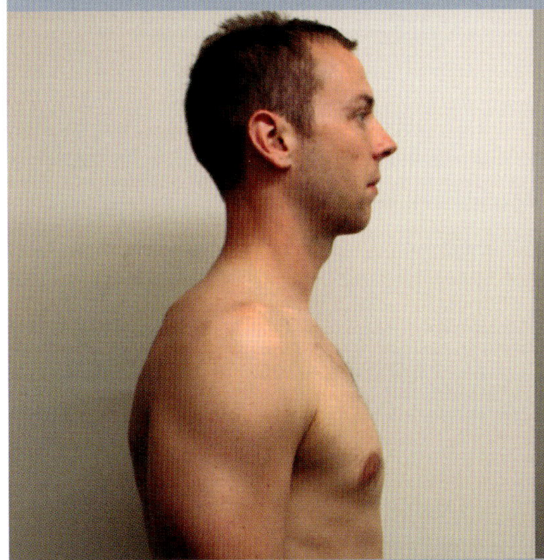

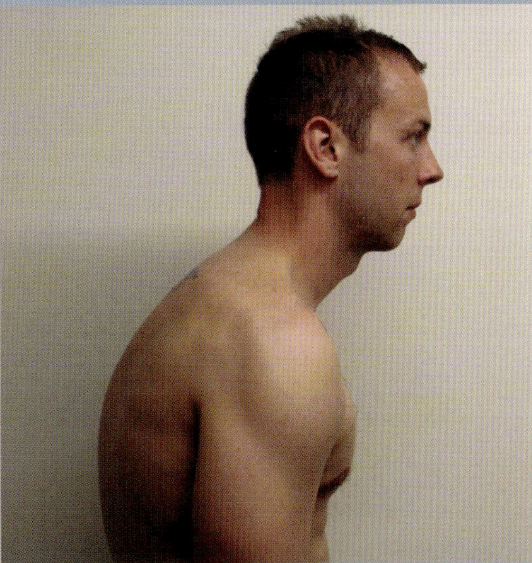

Figure 3.34
An increased curve of the upper back restricts the rotation of the scapula.

In order to re-establish movement, the muscles surrounding the shoulder blade can be treated with acupuncture, deep-tissue massage, or other therapies. Mobilising (encouraging movement) of the shoulder blade will also help correct abnormal movement of the shoulder blade.

Problems in the neck can both cause pain in the shoulder region due to referred pain and also change the movement patterns of the shoulder, causing ongoing shoulder pain. When treating the shoulder, it is imperative to assess the neck to ensure there is no major contribution to symptoms from the neck. The next chapter addresses the investigations that can be performed for neck pain.

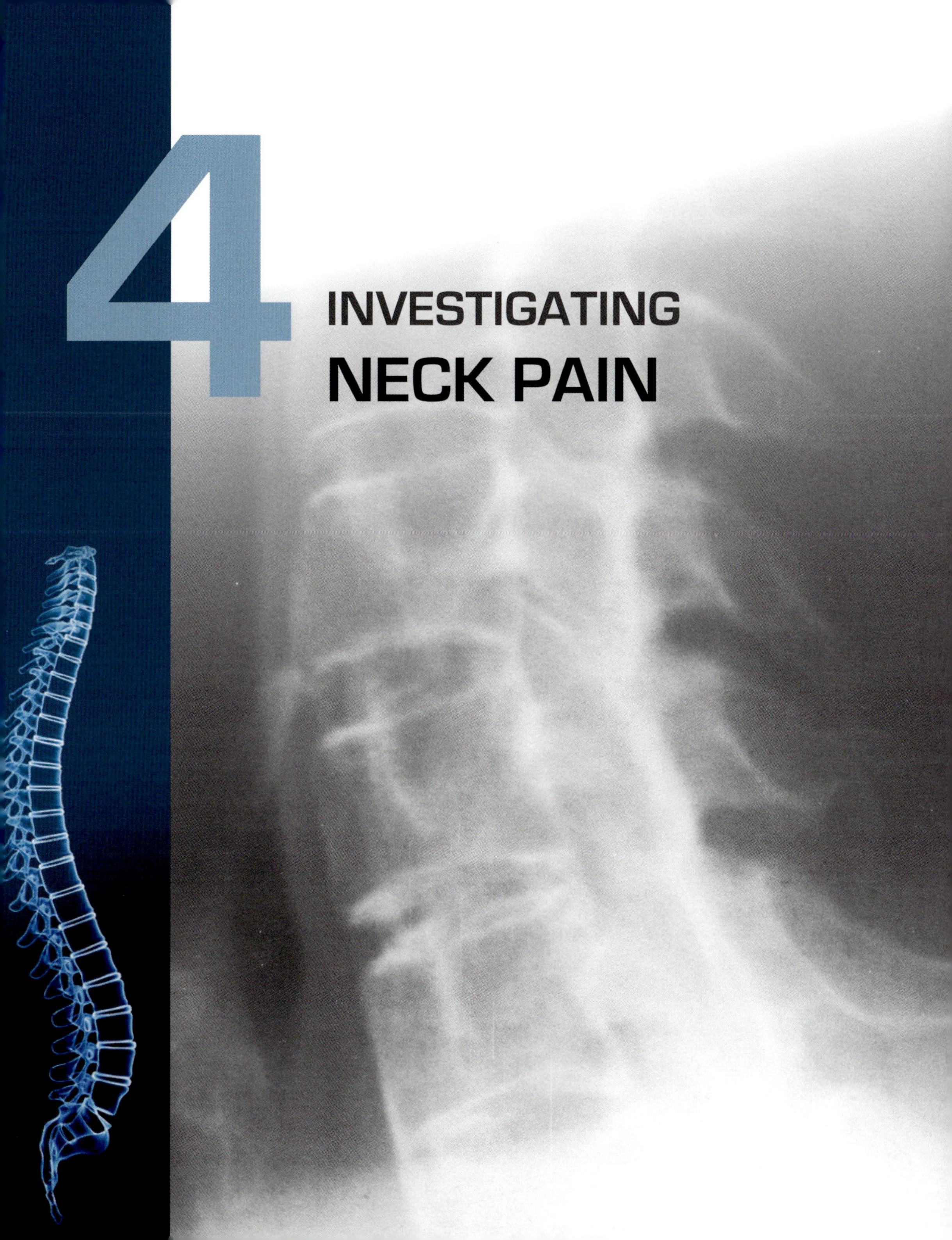

4 INVESTIGATING NECK PAIN

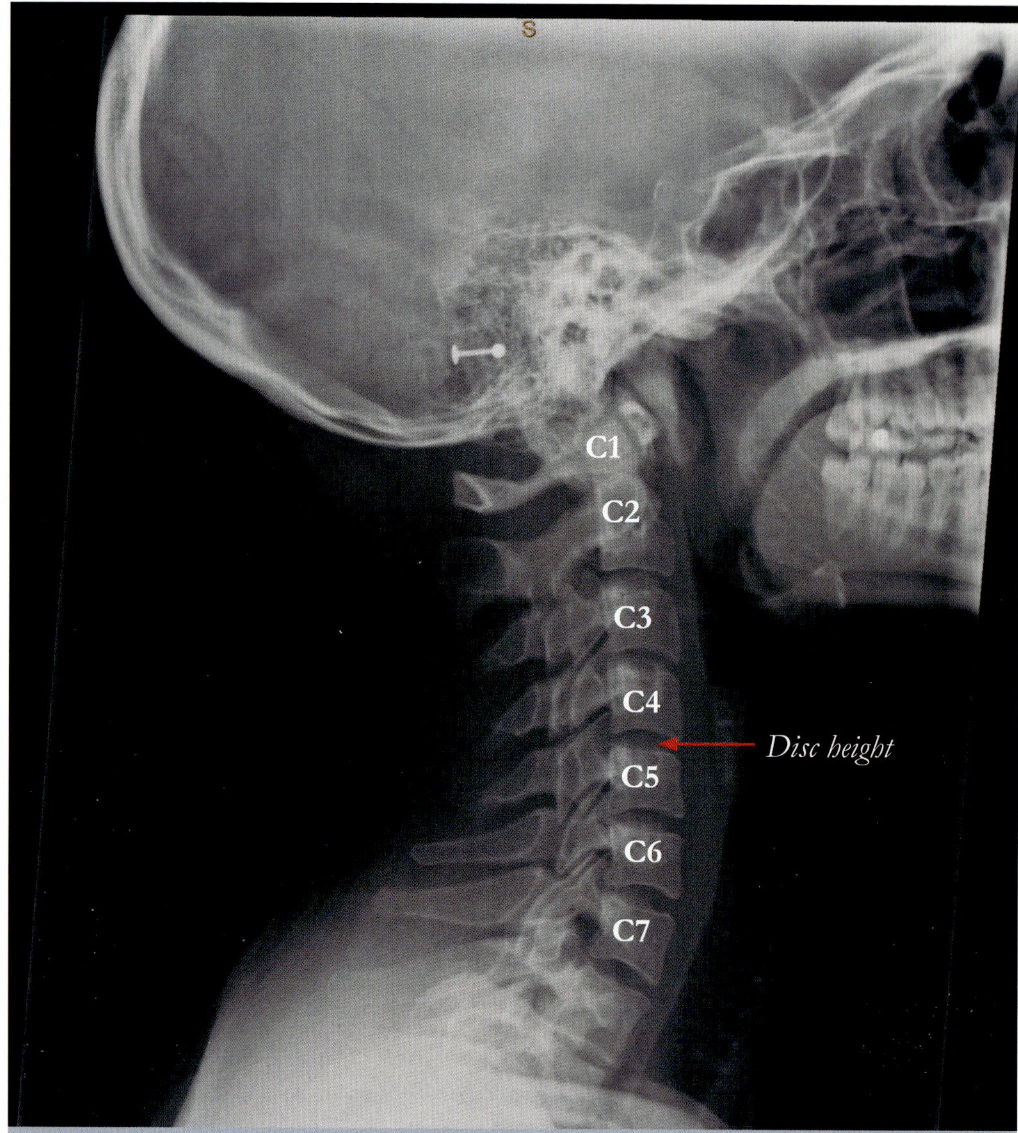

Figure 4.1
A neck X-ray can show the height of the disc (the gap between the vertebrae), fractures and other bone abnormalities.

Investigations are tests that can be performed for people suffering from neck pain to see what structure is damaged and might be causing pain. Although investigations are useful, they can pick up changes unrelated to pain, so must be interpreted with caution. The most common investigations performed for neck pain include X-ray, MRI scan, CT scan and bone scan.

X-ray

X-rays are useful for looking for fractures, especially for patients who have had trauma such as a fall or accident. X-rays may show variations present since birth (congenital variations), facet joint changes and wear and tear of bones. Figure 4.1 shows a neck X-ray. X-rays are stopped by solid objects but pass through objects such as discs that are mainly composed of water. Hence an X-ray shows the outline of the discs as a series of gaps between the bones. They are a useful first investigation as they give an appreciation of disc height as well as the shape of the neck.

CASE STUDY: *Philippa*

Philippa presented to my clinic with over 20 years' neck pain, which had spread to the back of her shoulder and was causing pins and needles in her right hand. Turning her neck, especially when driving, aggravated her pain the most. Sitting at a computer for long periods also aggravated her symptoms, and sleep had always been difficult as she could no longer find a comfortable position with respect to her neck.

Philippa had an X-ray performed seven years prior to my first consultation with her. This is seen in Figure 4.2 and shows subtle narrowing of the disc between the fifth and sixth vertebrae. A new X-ray taken seven years later showed the narrowing had increased along with the bony spurs surrounding the disc.

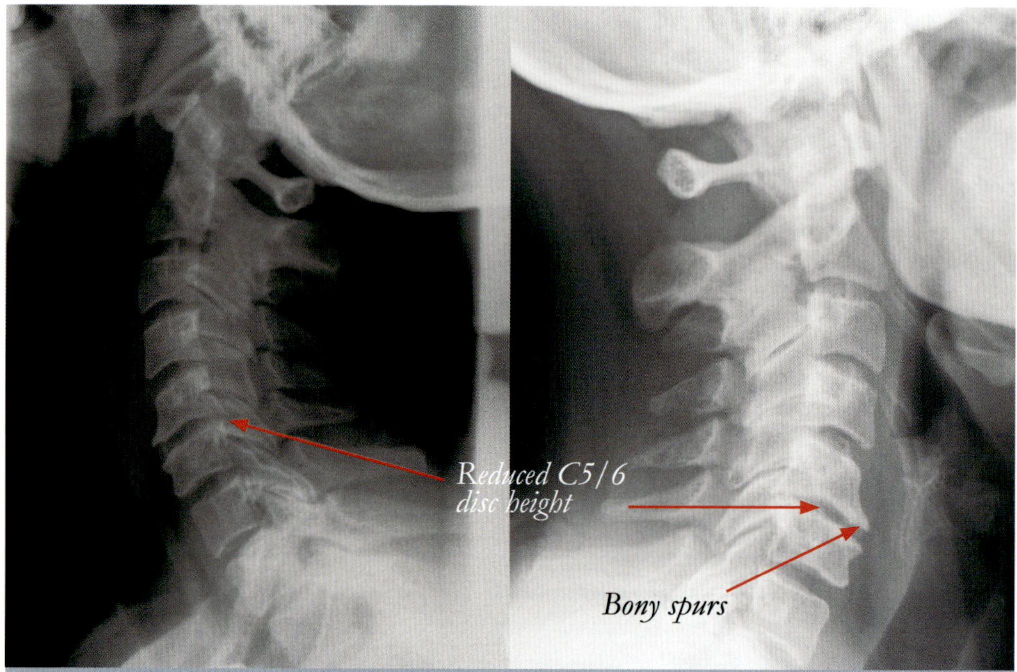

Figure 4.2
Philippa's X-ray of her neck in 2005 on the left with some narrowing of the C5/6 disc height. The X-ray on the right taken in 2012 shows increased narrowing of the disc and increased prominence of bony spurs surrounding the disc.

Magnetic resonance imaging

An MRI scan produces high-quality images of the soft tissues such as the disc. Unlike an X-ray that gives an appreciation of disc height, MRI scans show disc detail, such as how much fluid is present in the gel, whether there are tears in the ring ligament, disc height, and whether the disc is applying pressure to the nerves or spinal cord.

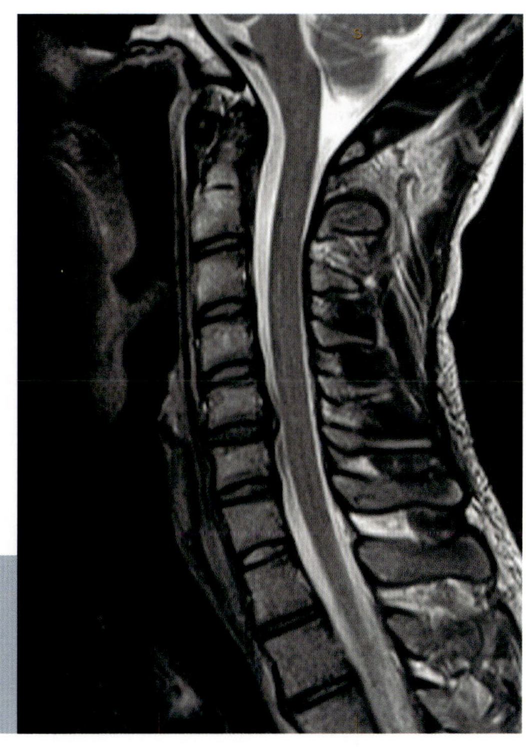

Figure 4.3

MRI scans show excellent soft tissue detail.

Magnetic resonance imaging scans use magnetic forces and do not subject the patient to radiation. A magnet is placed close to the body site being scanned and the scanner takes pictures of that part of the body, e.g. the shoulder, neck, and low back, and does not take a whole body scan. A disadvantage of MRI is that the scanner can be claustrophobic and emits a hammering noise.

CASE STUDY: *Kyle*

In December 2005, when Kyle was playing cricket, he ran onto the pitch and collided with his uncle's knee with his head in a bent position. He developed a sore neck and also pins and needles in his right fingers.

He was taken to the local hospital where X-rays were performed and reported as normal. He continued to suffer neck pain and headaches intermittently. An MRI scan performed seven years later confirmed a disc prolapse, shown between the fifth and sixth vertebrae of the neck.

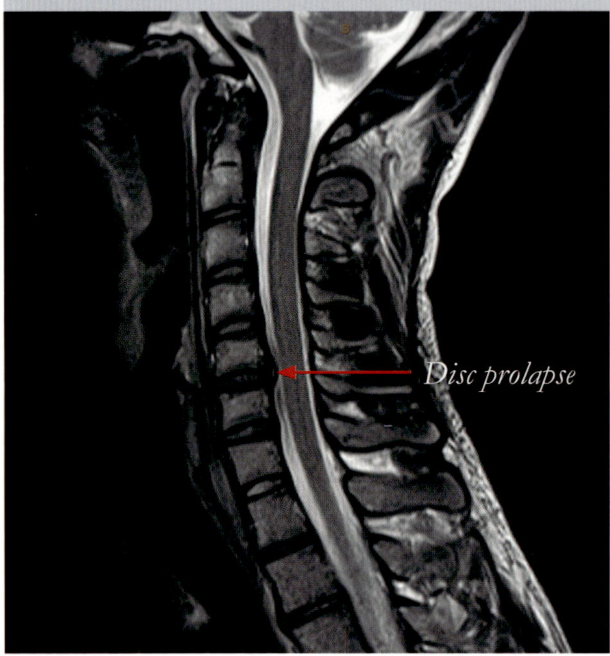

Figure 4.4
An MRI scan of the neck reveals a disc prolapse at C5/6 that was missed on an X-ray.

Computed tomography

A CT scan is like a super X-ray and gives much finer detail about bones. It is the best imaging technique when trying to figure out bony problems with precision. However, this precision comes with increased radiation, with one CT scan producing radiation equivalent to 5,000 chest X-rays. Figure 4.5 shows a CT scan image. CT scan images are excellent for determining the extent of osteophytes (bony spurs) surrounding narrow discs.

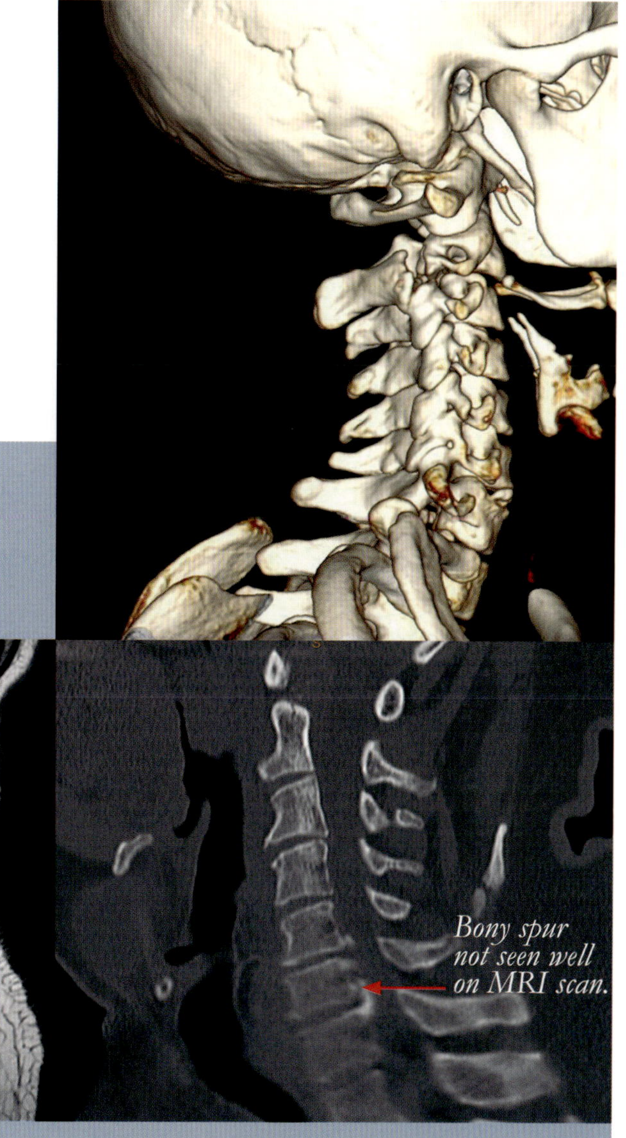

Figure 4.5

CT scan shows excellent bone detail.

Figure 4.6

The MRI scan on the left shows disc detail well and the CT scan on the right shows better detail of bony spurs.

Bone scan

A bone scan (Figure 4.7) is a nuclear bone scan that detects bone which is trying to heal. It is useful to diagnose bone cancers and detect stress fractures that do not show up on normal X-rays. The patient receives an injection containing a radioactive solution that is then detected by a camera. The patient is exposed to small amounts of radiation during this test.

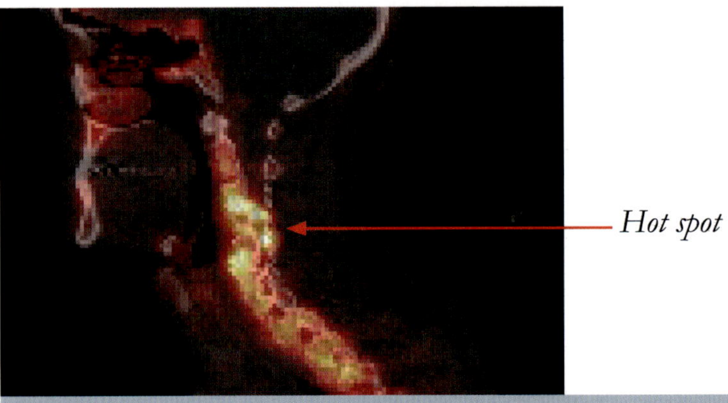

Figure 4.7
The image produced by a bone scan shows hotspots where bone is being irritated. This bone scan shows a hotspot (increased uptake of radioactive material) in the back of the neck.

Investigations may show abnormalities that have been present for a long time, and some that are irrelevant to the person's symptoms. Investigations need to be matched to the patient's story and examination to see if changes seen are relevant to the patient's pain complaint.

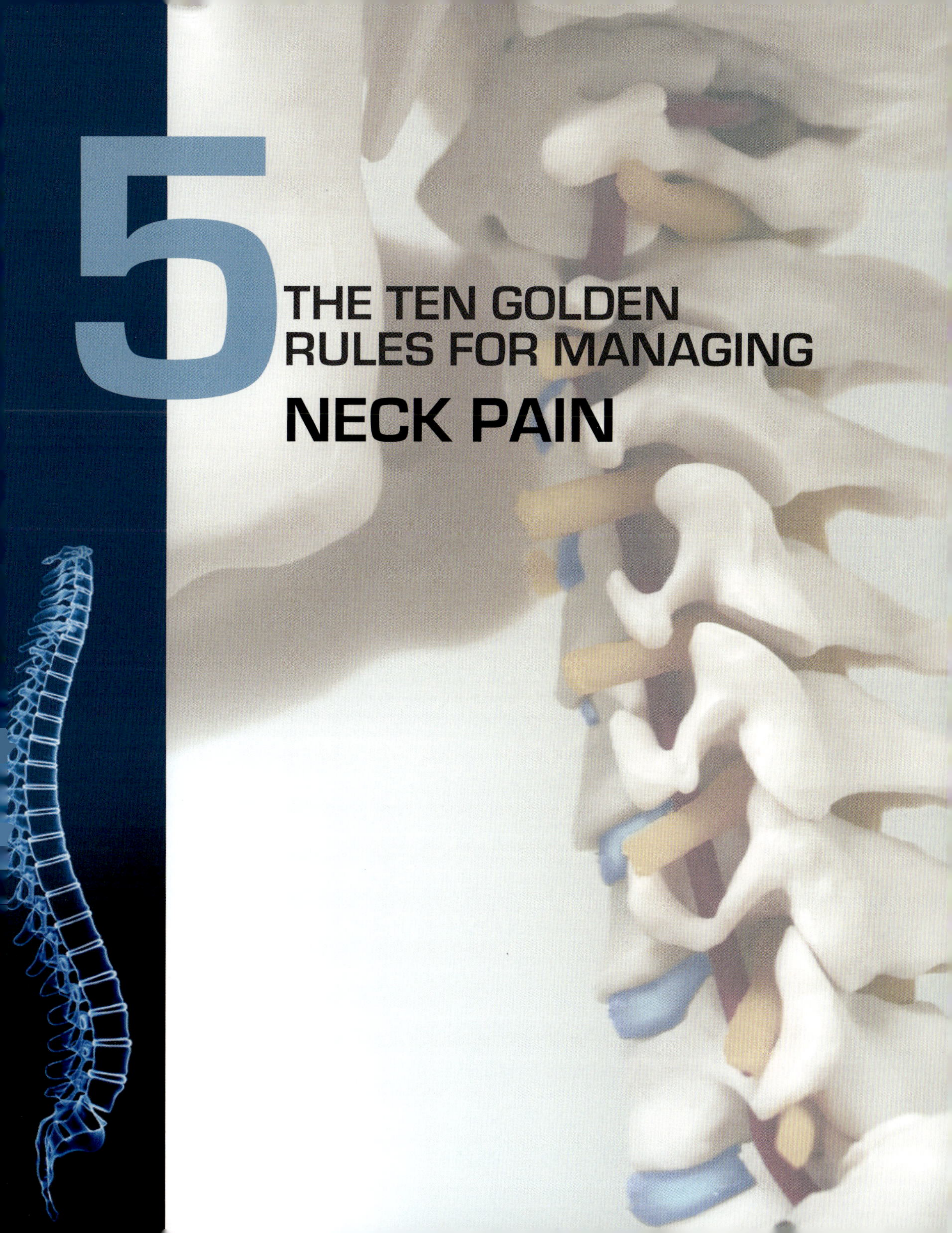

5 THE TEN GOLDEN RULES FOR MANAGING NECK PAIN

Managing neck pain

This chapter outlines the ten golden rules for managing neck pain. Pain is usually the result of pressure being generated by gravity. The advice is designed to reduce pressure on the discs of the neck, as they are the most common source of pain. Changing your posture to relieve pain involves reducing the gravitational force on the structure causing pain. The normal shape of the neck is curved when looking from the side. Maintaining this shape is essential to reducing forces on the discs in the lower neck.

1. Maintain the curve of the neck

The word lordosis refers to the curved shape of the neck as shown in Figure 5.1. The neck is not a straight column because the building blocks (vertebrae and discs) are not square. Instead the vertebrae and discs are wedge shaped and create this curve. If the vertebrae and discs were square and the spine were straight, problems would arise from the lifelong pressure generated, as the weight of the head and each vertebra would add directly to the pressure at the lower discs of the neck.

The beauty of the curved shape of the spinal column is that it allows pressure to be absorbed by increasing and decreasing the curve. So if you place a heavy container on your head, the curve would increase, reducing the height of the column. On unloading the heavy object, the spine would stretch again. Instead of crushing the bottom of the spine, pressure is relieved by the middle of the curve. The spine is essentially acting like a C-shaped spring that compresses when loading the spine and unwinds when taking load off the spine. Despite this design, however, damage to the discs still occurs, and the lower two levels (vertebrae) of the neck account for over 90% of the disc narrowing seen on X-rays and scans due to incorrect posture.

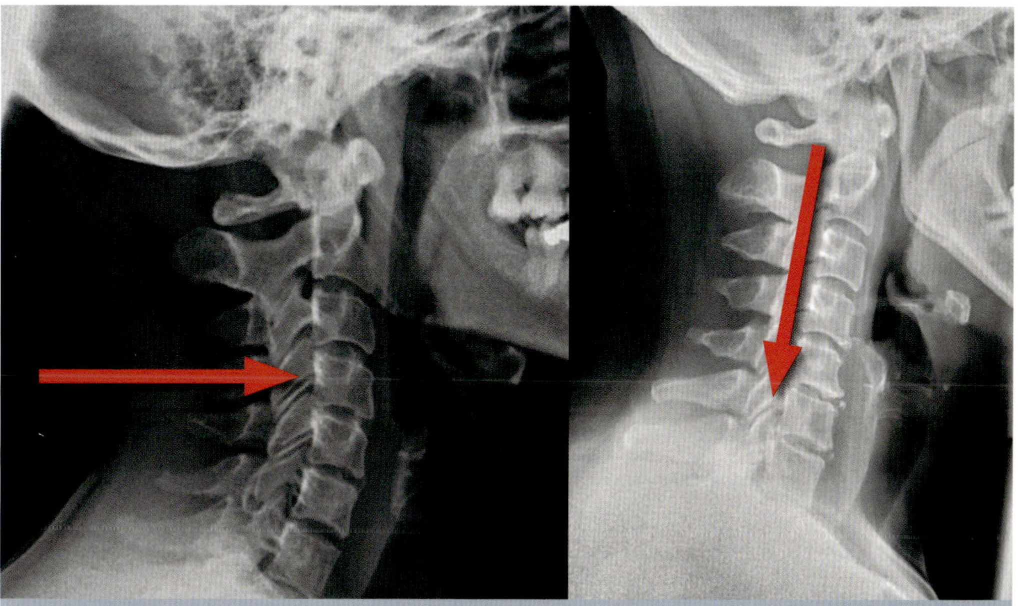

Figure 5.1

The backward C-shape curve of the neck on the left allows the weight of the head to be absorbed in the middle of the curve. A straight neck on the right causes the weight of the head to be directly transmitted to the lower neck discs.

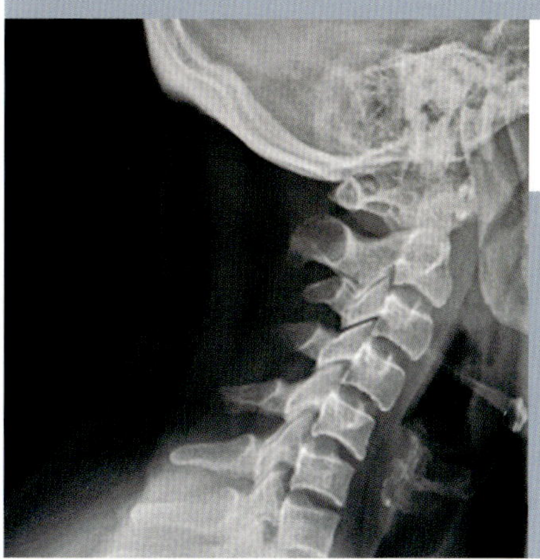

Figure 5.2

The backward C-shape neck has been reversed and increases pressure over the lower neck discs even more than a straight neck.

CASE STUDY: *Sam*

Sam was playing badminton, and, while going for a shot, developed neck pain as well as electrical symptoms of pins and needles, numbness and tingling down the left arm and hand. He worked as a podiatrist and would look down for long periods when treating people. His sleep was disturbed and he was waking with a stiff neck. An X-ray of the neck, as seen in Figure 5.3, shows the loss of a backward C-shape curve of the neck. There is a new curve in the opposite direction to the one it should follow. This places increased pressure on the discs of the lower neck. The curve has developed over many years due to looking down for long periods in his work as a podiatrist.

An MRI scan showed a disc prolapse. After following self-treatment to reduce the pressure on his lower neck and change some postures when working, he found his neck and arm pain reduced.

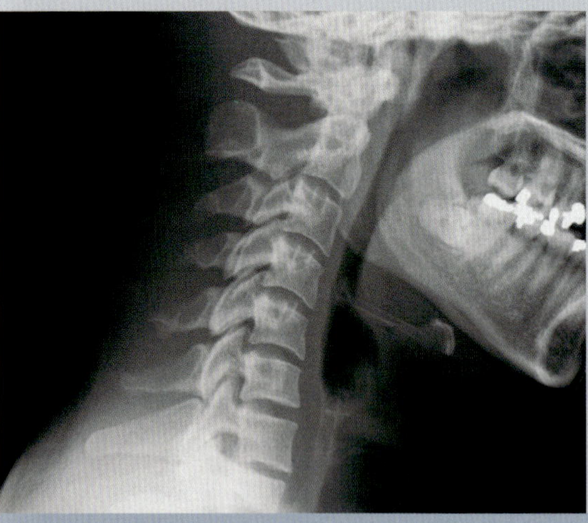

Figure 5.3
The X-ray showed a reversal of the normal shape curve of the neck that places extra pressure on the lower discs of the neck.

2. Avoid looking down for long periods

When the neck is placed into its normal curve shape, the pressure on the discs and the bones is at a minimum. However, if the curve is straightened by postures such as leaning forward for prolonged periods, the weight of the head and neck is constantly compressing the lower neck discs. In fact, for every 10 degrees you bend your neck forward, you double the pressure that the head exerts onto the lowest disc of the neck. Let's say your head weighs 5kg. If you are looking down at a 10-degree angle, the weight transferred through the lowest disc in the neck would be 10kg. If you flex your neck to 90 degrees, then your head would exert 45kg of pressure on the lowest disc. The disc will over the years become compressed with incorrect posture. The ring ligament may weaken, develop tears more easily and predispose you to episodes of neck pain from minor trauma.

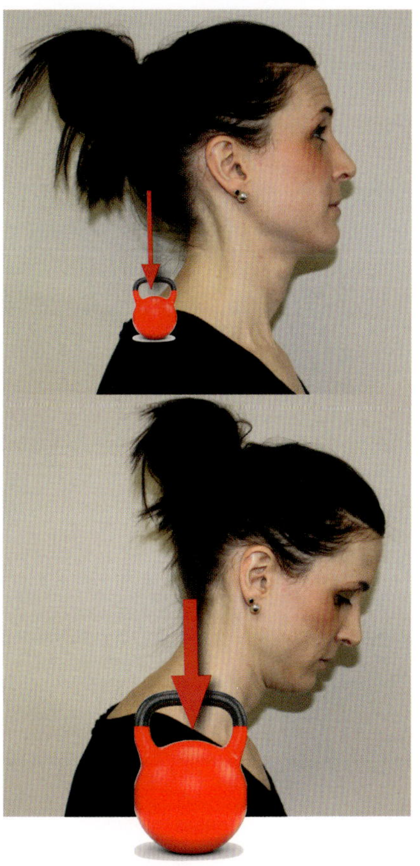

Figure 5.4
The force exerted by the head doubles with every 10 degrees of looking down, due to the change in the centre of gravity of the head. When looking straight ahead the weight of the head is approximately 5 kg. When looking 10 degrees down it increases the force to 10kg on the lower neck.

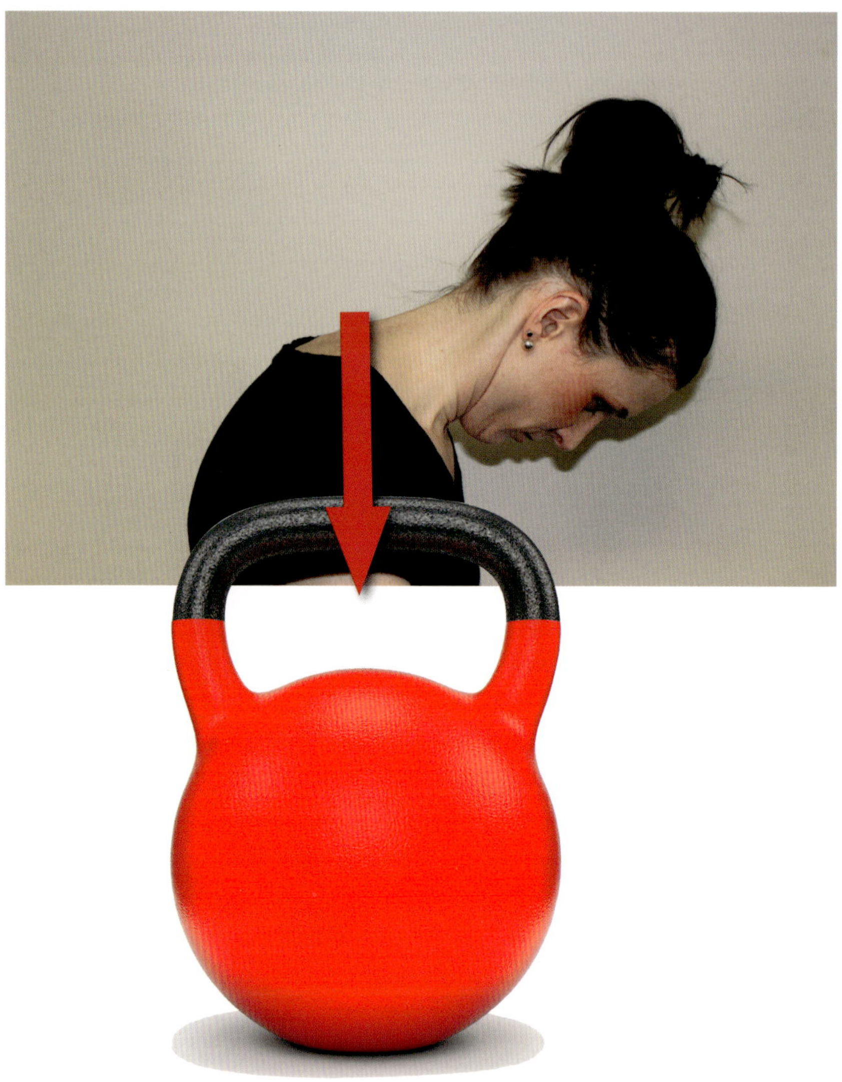

Figure 5.5
The force of the head on the lower neck increases to 45kg when looking down 90 degrees.

CASE STUDY: *Patricia*

Patricia worked as a pastry chef and cake decorator, and for many years spent her days working over a workbench, looking down. Six months before her consultation, she had a fall while playing netball and sprained her neck. The pain continued for some time, causing headaches and disturbed sleep. An X-ray was taken (Figure 5.7) that showed narrowing of the discs in the mid to lower neck with a straightening of the neck curve.

Patricia was told that years spent looking down at cakes was causing significant pressure on the base of the neck, leading to narrowing of the discs and aggravating her symptoms. Patricia performed traction exercises and modified her activities, often wearing a soft collar when working on cakes. Over several months her neck symptoms improved, and her headaches and sleep disturbance subsided. Despite the narrowing present in the neck, reducing the pressure alleviated her symptoms.

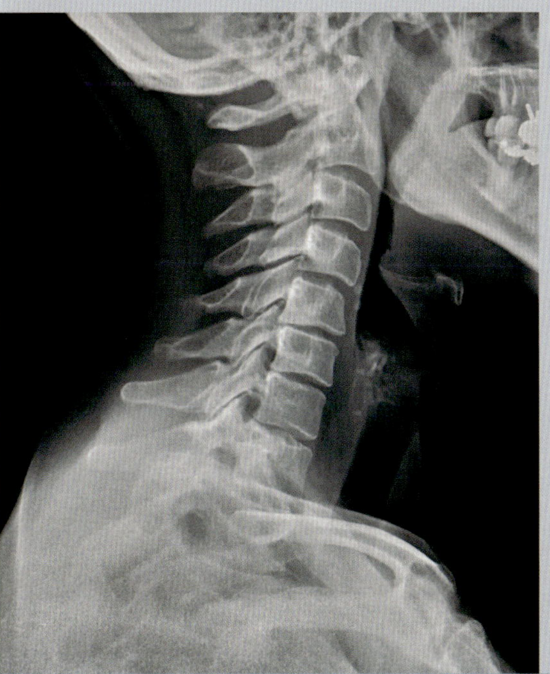

Figure 5.6
The discs in the lower neck are narrowed and the normal backwards C-shape curve of the neck has straightened.

3. Maintain good neck posture

Good posture is mostly concerned with the maintenance of this curve and reducing the force of the head that is transmitted through the lower neck. When you are sitting at the computer desk it is imperative that you should look straight ahead rather than look down. The screen needs to be raised, as shown in Figure 5.7. Sitting against the back of the chair helps to maintain the neck in good posture rather than leaning forward.

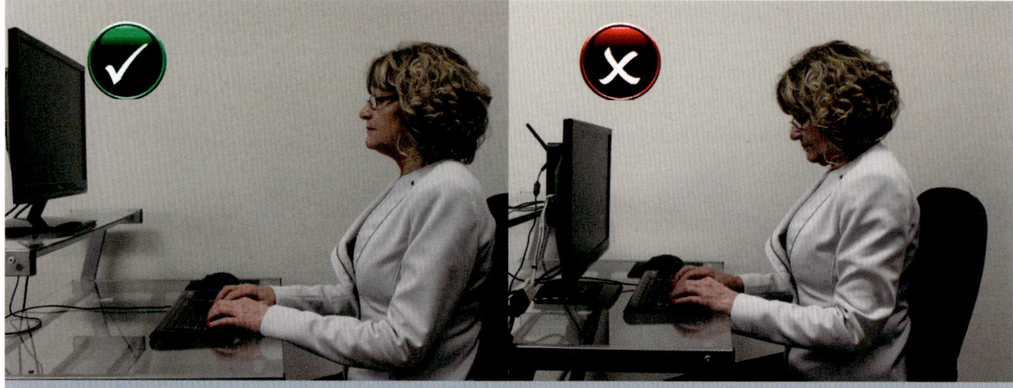

Figure 5.7
The left picture shows correct placement of a computer screen, with head upright and the back against the chair. The right picture shows an incorrect placement of screen and head, which increases the pressure placed on the lower neck discs.

When using a laptop, looking down will increase the pressure on the base of the neck and cause pain. If you use a laptop for more than five minutes, the laptop should be placed on a box to ensure the screen is at eye level, and a keyboard and mouse should be attached to the laptop as shown in Figure 5.8. When using a cellphone for long periods, looking down while messaging or going online (Figure 5.9) will increase pressure on the lower neck discs.

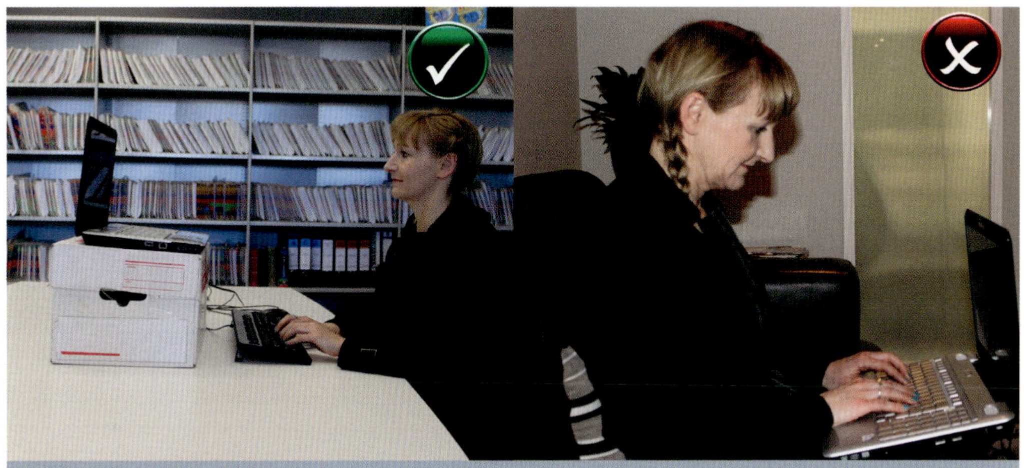

Figure 5.8

The left picture shows correct placement of a laptop computer, with head upright and the back against the chair. The right picture shows an incorrect placement of the laptop computer with low screen and flexed neck, which increases the pressure placed on the lower neck discs.

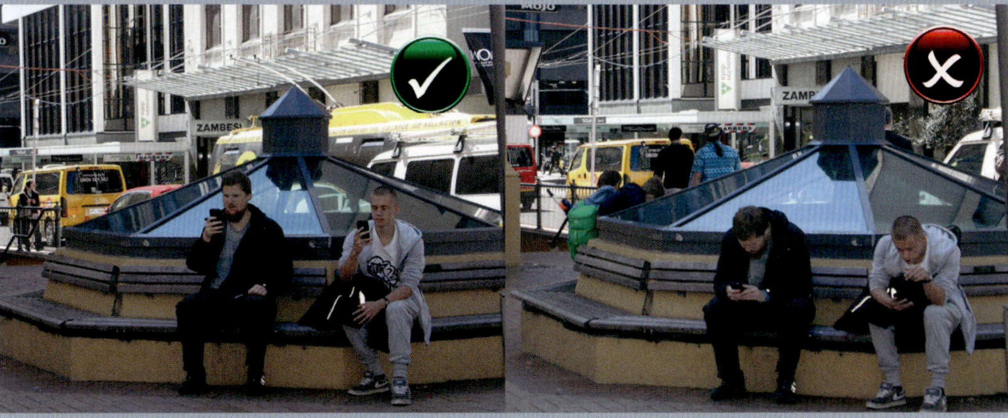

Figure 5.9

The posture on the left minimises the pressure on the lower neck while the right hand posture increases lower neck pressure.

Looking straight ahead will reduce pressure on the lower neck (Figure 5.9). When relaxing in the evening, reclining reduces the pressure that travels through the discs of the lower neck, as shown in Figure 5.10.

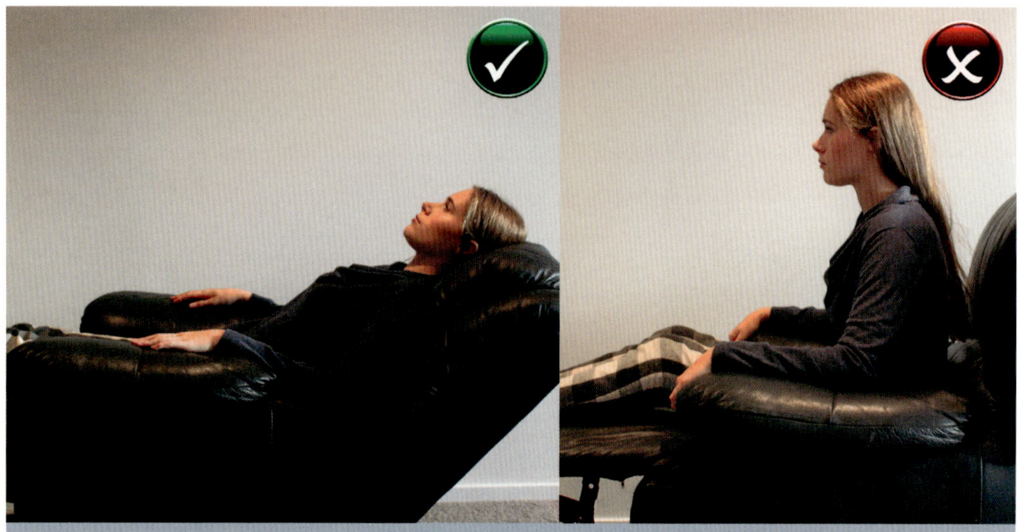

Figure 5.10
Reclining as shown on the left reduces the pressure on the lower neck discs. Sitting upright increases pressure on the lower neck discs.

If you enjoy reading, bring the book up to eye level rather than look down on it for long periods, as seen in Figure 5.11. Reading on your front, as shown in Figure 5.12, reduces pressure on the lower discs of the neck. If you write for long periods, a sloping desk (Figure 5.13) is useful, as it reduces the amount you need to bend your neck. Crafts such as sewing and cross-stitch often require you to look down for several hours at a time and are a common source of neck pain. It is important to take regular breaks and also to wear a soft collar when performing these activities to ensure you do not place constant pressure on the base of the neck.

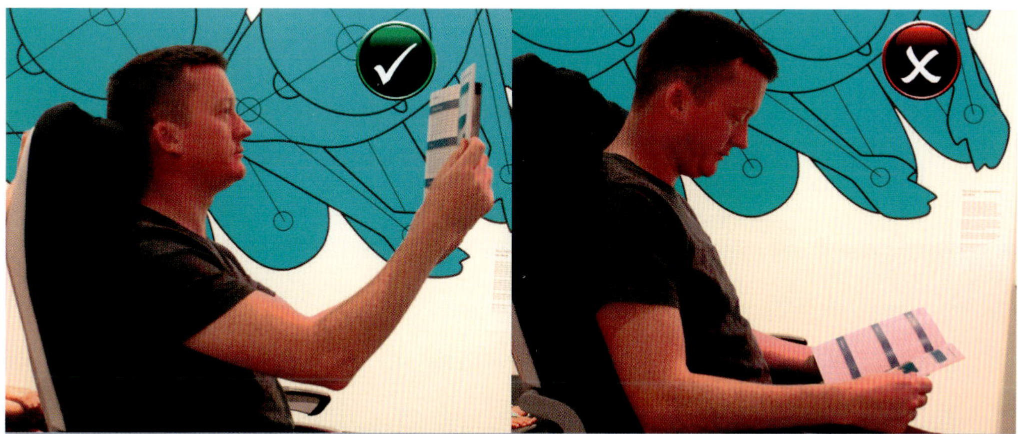

Figure 5.11

When reading, bending the head creates increased pressure on the lower neck leading to compression of the lower neck. Reading with the book raised reduces pressure on the lower neck. Sometimes you may need a copyholder or easel to maintain good posture while reading.

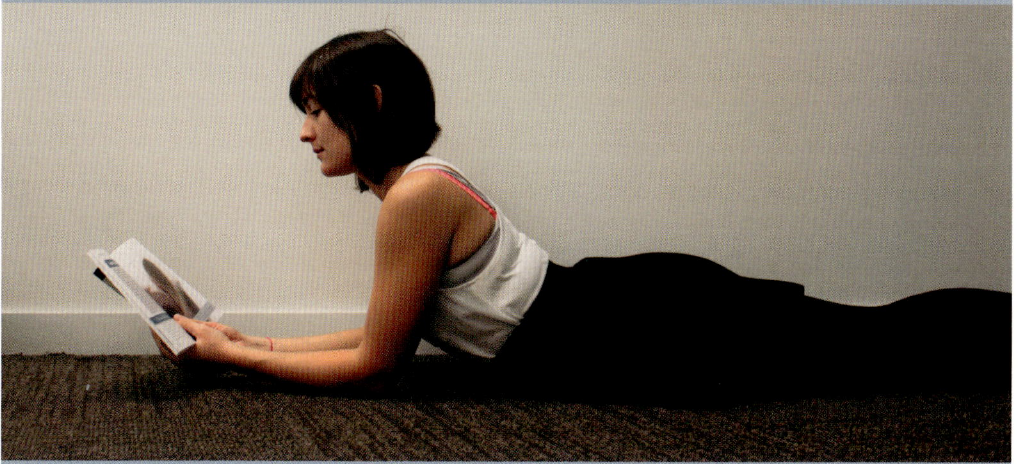

Figure 5.12

Reading on your front can reduce disc pressure in the lower neck.

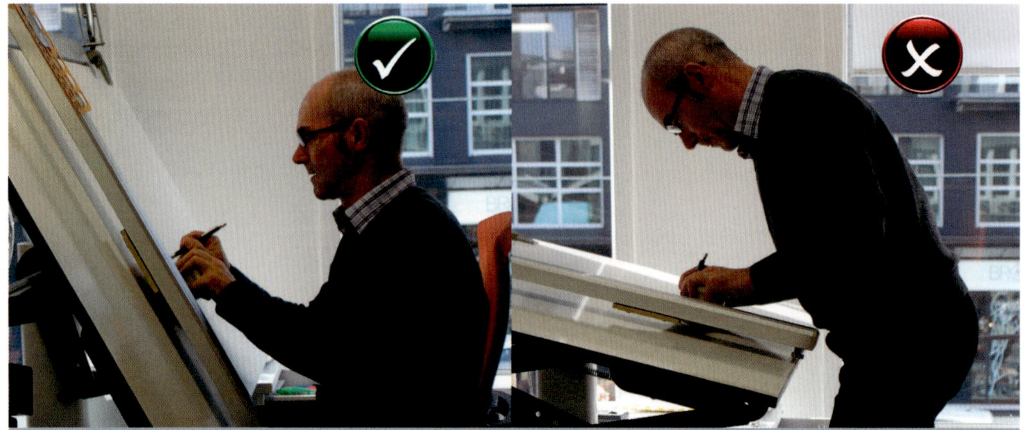

Figure 5.13

When writing, a sloping desk will reduce pressure placed on the lower neck discs.

CASE STUDY: *Donna*

Donna, a 35 year old woman, was experiencing neck pain, shoulder pain, and pins and needles in her neck and left arm. Examination revealed tenderness over the neck muscles and arm muscles, as well as a restricted range of motion of the neck. Donna first consulted me in 2007.

The X-ray in Figure 5.14 revealed a straight neck with loss of the normal curved shape as well as narrowing of the disc between the fifth and sixth vertebrae. An MRI scan of the neck showed three big slipped discs. When shown to a medical colleague, he stated that, in his opinion, it was almost certain this patient would have required surgery.

Donna enjoyed cross-stitch, a hobby that involves looking down at a tapestry canvas for long periods of time. I advised her she needed to stop cross-stitch and other activities which require looking down for long periods, as for every 10 degrees she flexed her neck, the pressure of the head doubled on the lower neck and the increased pressure squeezed discs slightly further. She was placed in a soft collar and advised to perform traction of the neck by placing her head off the bed. Her muscles were treated with a combination of acupuncture and saline injections, and over two months her symptoms improved.

After the first six months, Donna's symptoms settled almost completely, and she modified her activity, including giving up cross-stitch. She has not experienced a significant relapse of pain over the past seven years. She also continues to perform traction over the bed regularly to avoid relapses.

This casc illustrates the improvement that can occur even in the most severe disc prolapses by changing posture to reduce pressure on the neck and performing traction. Moreover, improvement can be sustained for many years with the right advice. This case also illustrates the difference between an X-ray and MRI scan. The X-ray (Figure 5.14) showed some changes but did not show the large disc prolapses present at several levels. If nerve symptoms are present, an MRI scan (Figure 5.15) is an excellent choice of investigation for the neck.

C5/6 disc height narrowing

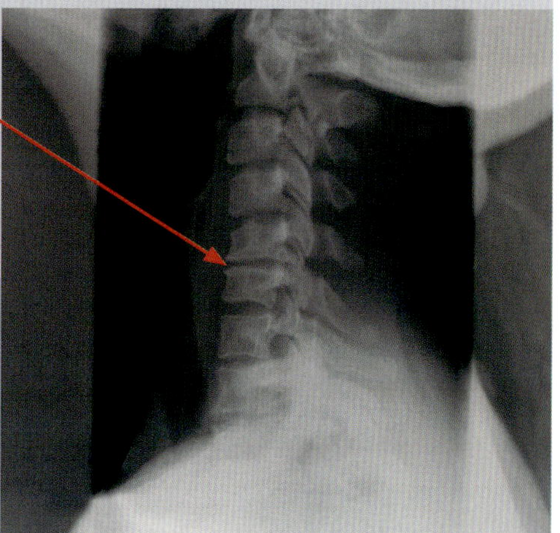

Figure 5.14
The neck X-ray displays both loss of the curve and also narrowing of the disc between the fifth and sixth vertebrae.

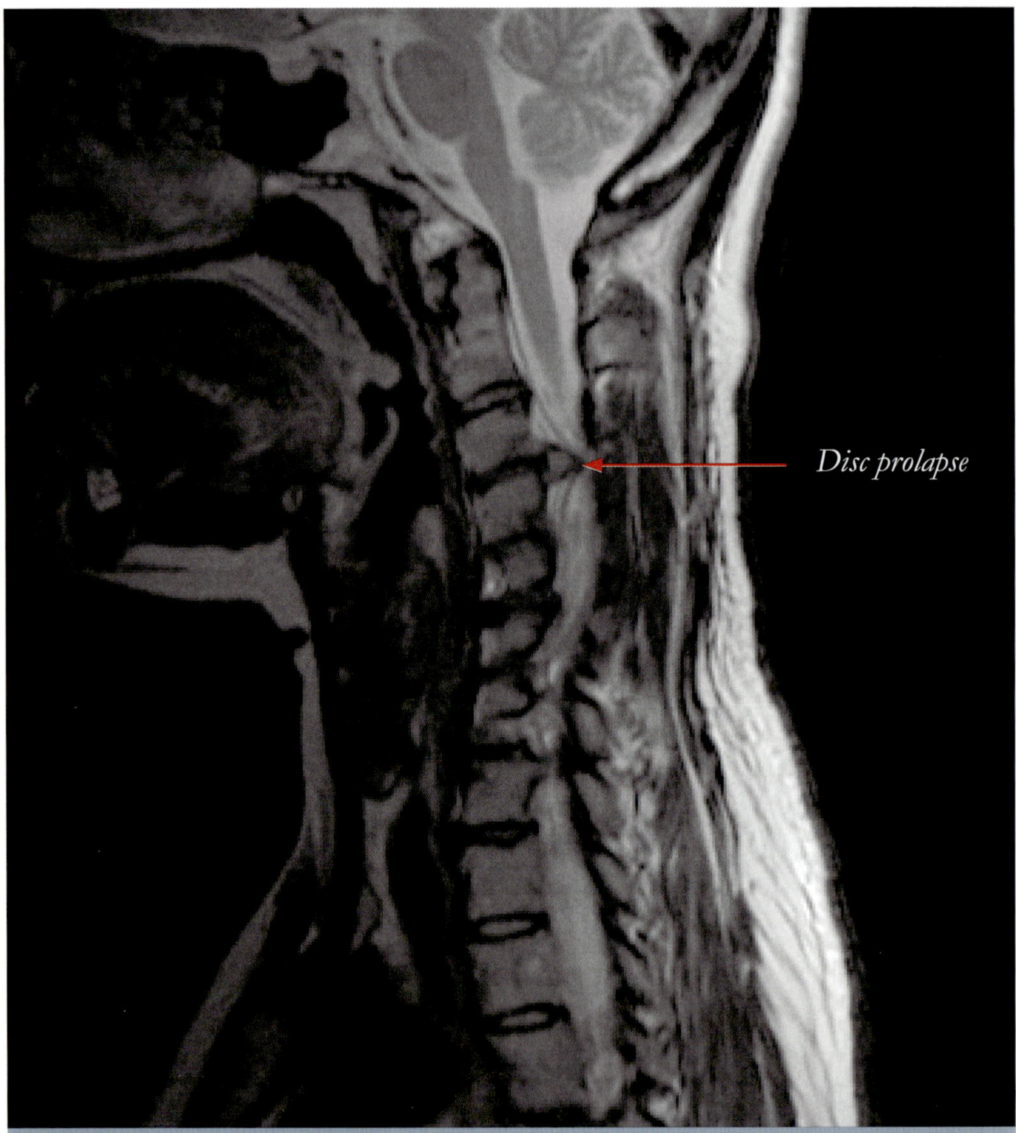

Figure 5.15

The MRI scan displays a reversed curve of the neck and a very large disc prolapse between the third and fourth vertebrae.

4. *Change postures frequently*

When sitting upright for prolonged periods it is good to get up and down off the seat regularly. Over time, the head weighs heavily on the neck, fluid is removed from the disc and travels to adjacent vertebrae, and the ability of the disc to absorb pressure reduces. Therefore, after 10 to 20 minutes, pressure increases at the base of the neck when you sit upright, especially when sitting still. Getting up and down from the desk every 30 minutes will help reduce constant disc pressure.

5. *Ensure good sleeping posture*

If you have suffered from neck pain, you are likely to have tried several pillows to reduce neck pain and stiffness. If your pillow puts the position of the neck into an incorrect posture, neck pain can increase during the night, either waking you during the night or causing neck stiffness or headache upon waking. As discussed earlier, pressure on the discs creates electricity that is relayed to the brain as pain. As pressure builds, electricity builds and when a certain amount of electricity is generated, pain is experienced.

The disc is sandwiched between two bones, and if the neck is bent while you are lying on your side, part of the disc will feel increased pressure, while the other side will have reduced pressure. When a disc is damaged it does not absorb pressure as well, and pressure on the disc and adjacent vertebrae can result in pain. When sleeping on your side your neck should remain straight, as shown in Figure 5.16, rather than having a pillow that is too thin or too thick.

If you have a soft bed, your shoulder will sink into the bed and you may need a narrow pillow. However, if your bed is hard then you may need a thicker pillow to maintain a straight neck when lying on your side. If you have broad shoulders, you may also require a thicker pillow. Trial and error is often necessary to get the right pillow for your neck.

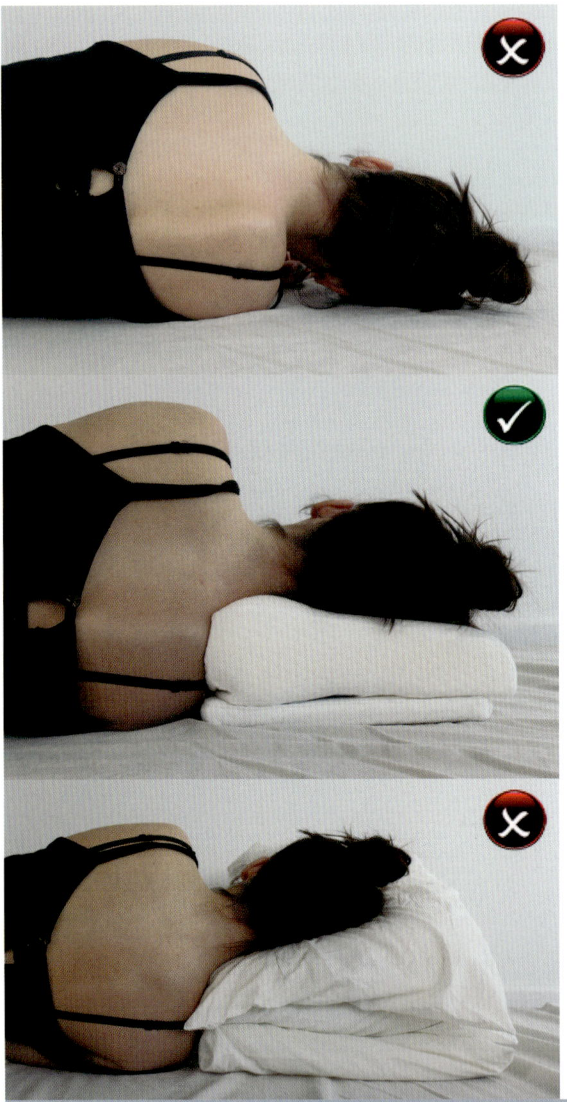

Figure 5.16

When sleeping on the side, the neck needs to remain straight to maintain the minimum pressure on the neck discs. The space between the bed and the head needs to be filled up by the pillow.

A memory foam pillow is helpful for around half of all patients with neck pain. Once you sink into a memory foam pillow, you often do not move, as it moulds your neck and head. Many pillows are contoured to fit your shoulder, head and neck shape in order to maintain a straight neck when lying on your side. If your sleep is disturbed with neck pain and stiffness during the night or in the morning, you should experiment with different pillows until you find one that reduces neck pain and stiffness at night.

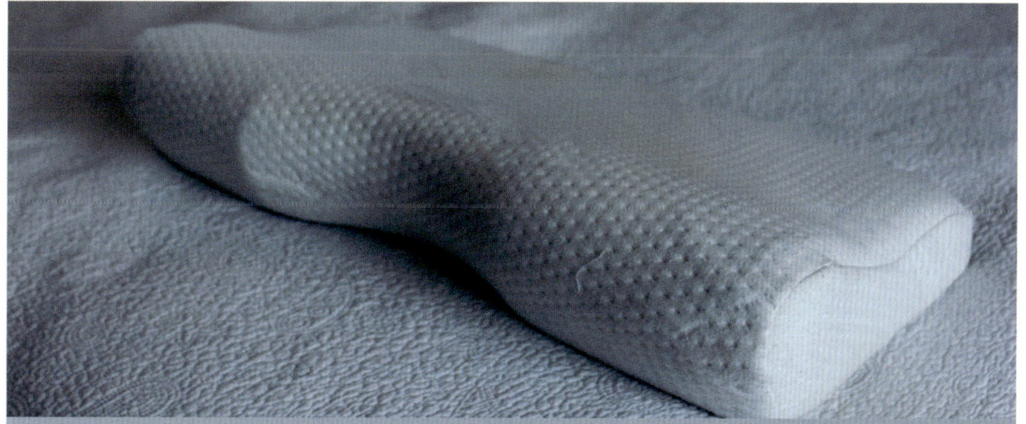

Figure 5.17
A memory foam pillow with a curved shape from the side profile and a curved shape in the front to accommodate the shoulder. This shape helps the neck stay in a straight position, reducing disc pressure, when you are lying on your side.

6. Wear a soft collar when looking down.

Pressure on the discs can aggravate pain and also aggravate nerve compression, so using a neck collar to reduce pressure on the discs is likely to help symptoms if used judiciously. I have prescribed soft collars to patients for many years with excellent results in improving pain. Most patients do not need to wear a soft collar after their neck pain improves over three months.

A soft collar can help neck pain by improving the shape of the neck as well as absorbing pressure that would normally fall on the discs at the lower neck. Soft collars for the neck are worthwhile trying as they are cheap compared to many therapies and directly target the site of pain. Pressure of the head on the neck discs causes pain, and for every 10 degrees you look down, you double the pressure exerted by your head.

Wearing a soft collar when performing activities that require you to look down, such as cooking, reduces the pressure that falls on the neck. Instead of the pressure being relayed to the discs of the lower neck, the pressure is absorbed by the foam at the front of the collar.

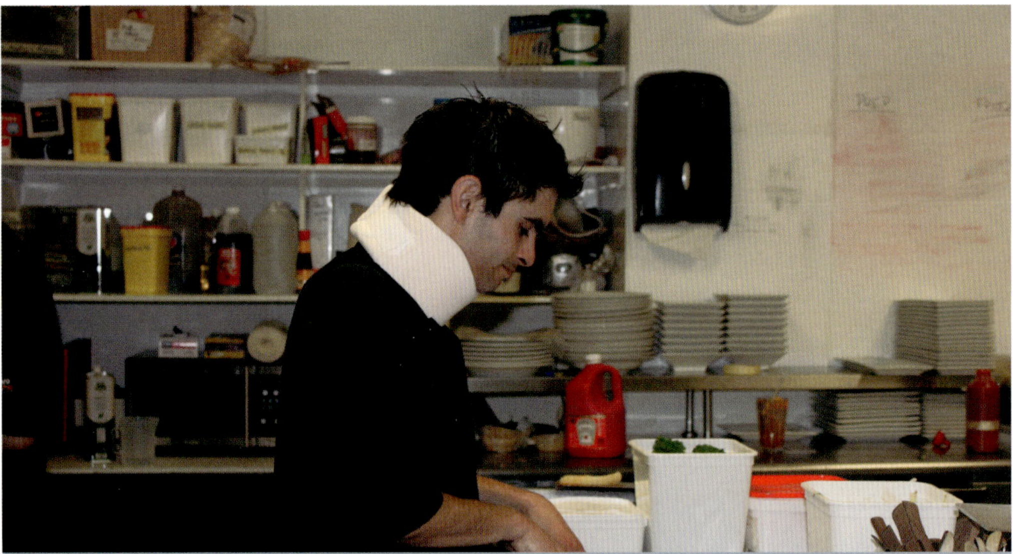

Figure 5.18

Wearing a soft collar while performing activities that require you to look down for long periods, such as cooking, can help reduce pain by limiting the pressure absorbed by the neck discs and instead transferring the pressure to the foam at the front of the collar.

The soft collar can be worn for several hours at a time with little risk of weakening muscles. People are often told that wearing a neck collar may weaken the muscles, but in fact it is pain that causes muscle weakness. Wearing a collar often helps pain, and that, in turn, improves the strength of the neck muscles.

People with severe neck pain can wear semi-rigid collars (Figure 5.19) as can people who experience troublesome arm symptoms from the neck. Studies have shown that semi-rigid collars are as useful as operations for disc prolapse or other physical therapies in the long term. I will often trial a semi-rigid collar with people who do not respond to the soft collar, especially for those who are taking longer to settle and are distressed by their symptoms.

A study of over 200 patients with recent onset disc prolapse of the neck showed a semi-rigid collar and rest was very effective in relieving pain and disability[4]. Patients wore the semi-rigid collar for approximately four hours a day in the first three weeks and then reduced the time it was worn.

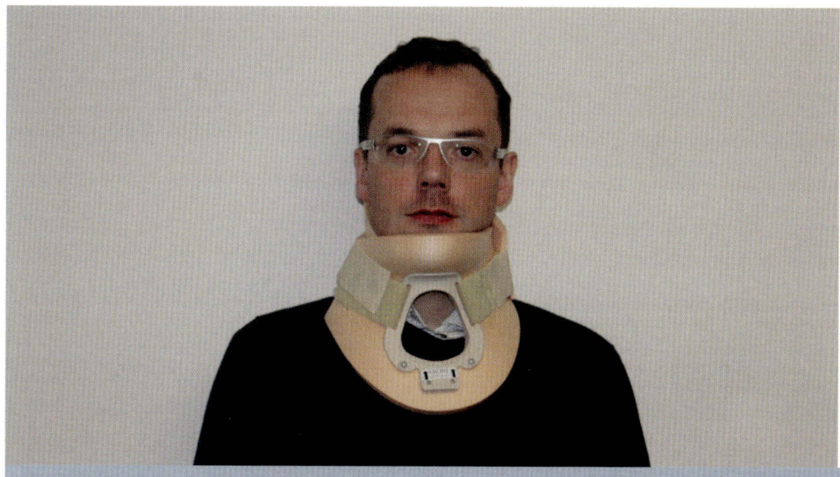

Figure 5.19
A semi-rigid collar allows less movement of the neck and reduces pressure on the discs. It should not be worn for more than three to four hours a day as stiffness of the neck may develop.

A semi-rigid collar transfers the weight of the head off the lower neck, relaying the weight to the shoulder regions. Once pressure is reduced on the discs, they can start the process of healing and over time become less sensitive to pressure. For patients not responding to a soft collar and for those who have a disc prolapse, the semi-rigid collar can often be very useful to alleviate pain.

7. Try traction therapies

The size and weight of the head pressing on the base of the neck can create pain, easing the pressure on the base of the neck is likely to help with the pain. Traction therapy reduces the pressure on the neck from the head, essentially by pulling the head away from the neck using a variety of devices, as shown in Figures 5.20 and 5.21. Several studies have shown traction of the neck can help both neck pain and headache. The simplest form of traction

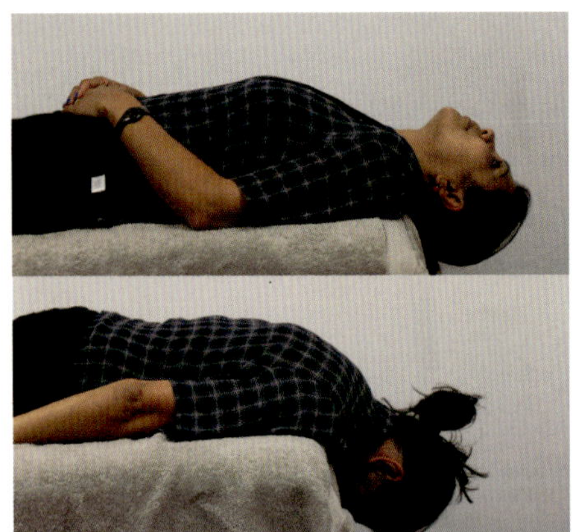

Figure 5.20
Traction can be performed as simply as lying on the bed with your head hanging off the end. This can be performed lying on your back, as shown, or lying on your front if lying on your back creates neck, shoulder or arm pain.

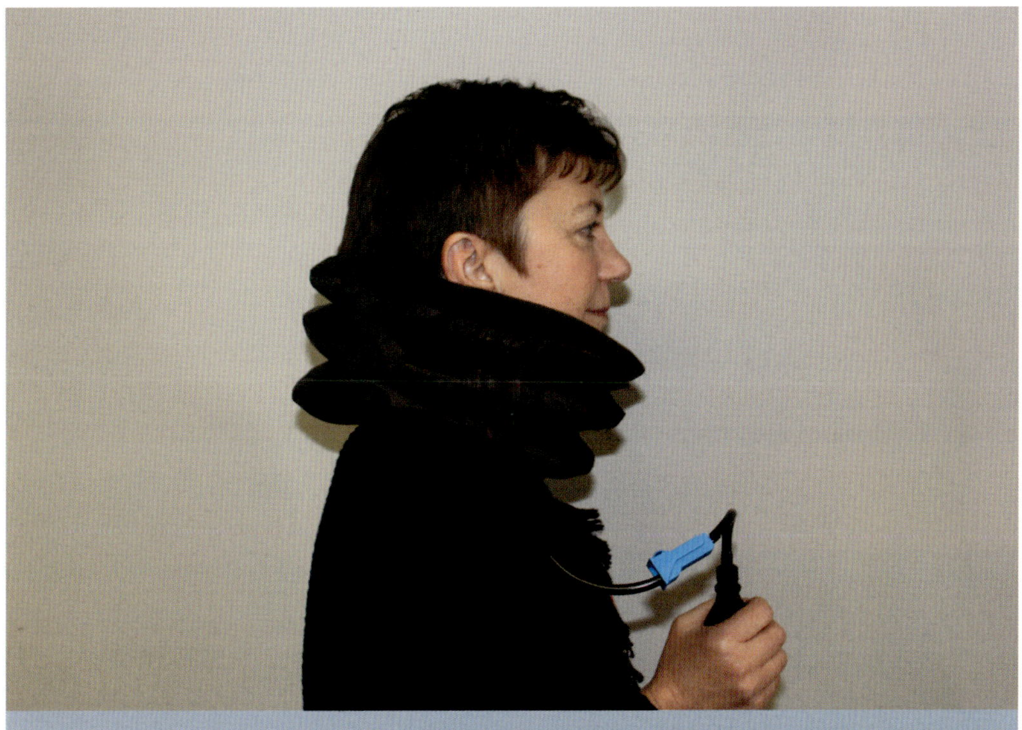

Figure 5.21
This traction collar fits around the neck with Velcro straps. By pumping the blood pressure cuff type device, the user can ensure that the collar lifts the weight of the head off the neck, creating traction of the neck discs.

that requires no equipment is hanging your head off the edge of a bed while lying on it (Figure 5.20). Once you are positioned with your head hanging off the bed, breathe gently for two minutes. Get up for 20 seconds, and repeat for another two minutes. This exercise can be performed lying on your back or front. When performed lying on your back this may improve the backward C-shaped curve of the neck, so this should be tried first. If lying on your back increases neck, arm or shoulder pain, lie on your front with the head off the bed. This will equally pull the head away the neck and reduce pressure on the neck, thereby reducing neck pain. Although the pressure is removed only temporarily, this manoeuvre allows fluid to return to the disc for several hours. This exercise should be performed at least twice a day, when waking and before going to sleep, but can also be performed during the day as often as needed.

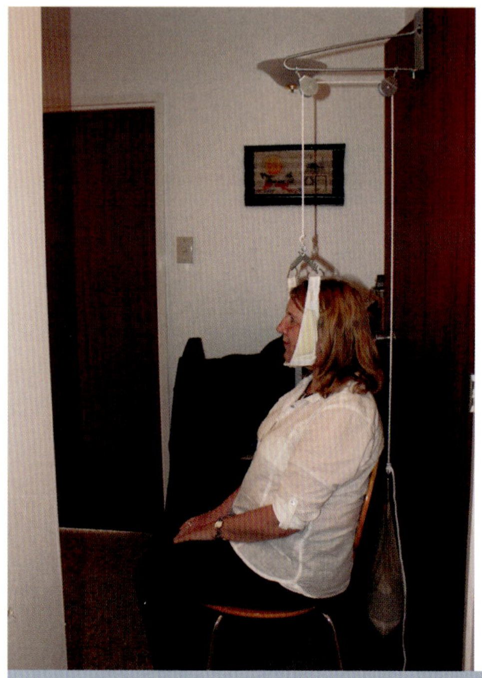

Figure 5.22
A neck traction device is shown that uses the door and weights hanging from a pulley.

In 1960, a study of neck traction of 2,000 people with chronic headaches arising from a neck injury showed that 80% were completely relieved of their symptoms[5]. Traction of the neck results in reduced muscle spasm surrounding the neck. Studies measuring electrical activity within the muscle after six weeks of traction have shown a 71% reduction in electrical activity in the muscles of the neck[6].

A study looked at MRI scans of the neck for people with prolapsed discs[8]. Traction with an air-inflated neck device showed a reduction of the disc prolapse when traction was applied. During traction, all volunteers and 21 out of 29 patients had a substantial increase in the length of the cervical vertebral column. The disk prolapse was completely resolved in three patients and partially reduced in 18 patients.

A study performed in 2008 measured disc height by comparing MRI scans before and after traction. They found that disc height increased by an average 19%, together with an improved range of motion, after traction[9].

Traction is by far the best initial management for neck pain.

In 2013 I started prescribing a collar that provides traction of the neck similar to a blood pressure cuff, as shown in Figure 5.21. This device fits around the neck with Velcro and is pumped up via the hand pump. The collar inflates, lifting the head away from the neck. This simple and inexpensive device can be used for five minutes several times a day. I advise people to take it to work and perform traction at morning tea and lunch to alleviate the pressure that builds up when sitting at the computer over time. Many patients found the collar to be very effective.

8. Maintain the muscle strength of the neck

When a person develops neck pain from the discs, signals are sent to the surrounding muscles that causes muscle spasm and develop into muscle knots called myofascial trigger points. The muscle knots are very tender when pressure is applied.

The muscle knots remain for a long time and can themselves start generating pain when stretched or pressed. They can also be responsible for a feeling of stiffness. Therapies such as deep tissue massage, stretching, acupuncture needling or injections can target these muscle knots and are discussed in the next chapter.

Performing exercises with an elastic band such as shown in Figure 5.23 will help stretch muscles and maintain muscle tone. A study of 180 female office workers[12] with an average of eight years of neck pain found neck pain reduced by more than 66% over 12 months. Furthermore neck muscle strength and range of motion increased while the intake of painkillers and visits to health professionals reduced markedly.

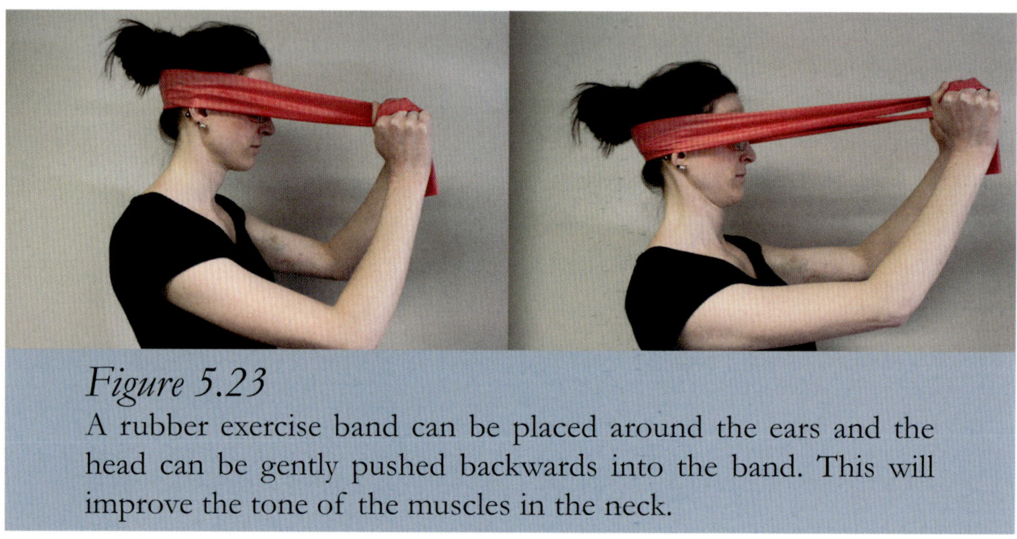

Figure 5.23
A rubber exercise band can be placed around the ears and the head can be gently pushed backwards into the band. This will improve the tone of the muscles in the neck.

9. Restore the curve in your neck

The spine is like plasticine; it takes the shape you give it. The neck normally has a backward C-shape curve (lordosis), however if you hold postures where you are flexing your neck for long periods such as looking down or bending forward when at the computer, then the backward C-shape curve can become straight or reversed. Both shapes increase loading on the lower neck discs and increase the chances of developing neck pain.

If an X-ray shows your curve is straightened or reversed, then using a rolled up towel and placing it under your neck while lying on the ground for five to 10 minutes a day should slowly restore your backward C-shape curve. The roll can be small to start with and then gradually be increased in size. Any soft cylindrical object such as a paper towel roll or small plastic drink bottle can be used for this manoeuvre. The curve may take six to 12 months to become restored so this exercise needs to be performed over several months rather than a few weeks.

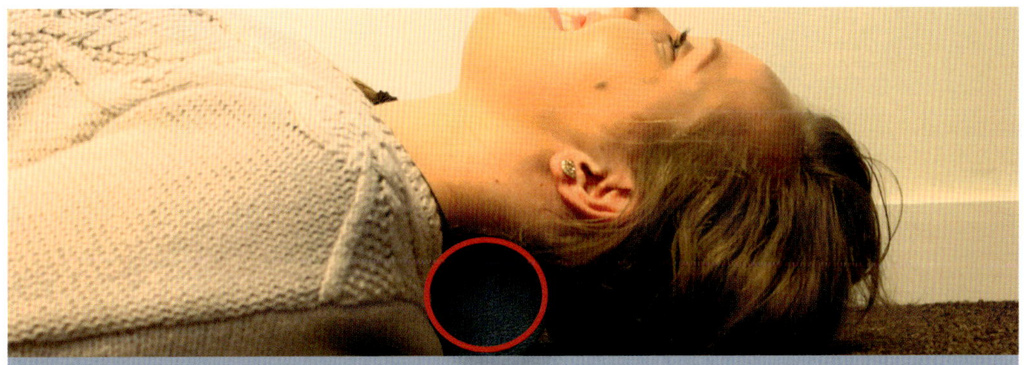

Figure 5.24
The left hand X-ray shows a normal backward C-shape neck (lordosis). The middle X-ray shows a straight neck and the right X-ray shows a reversal of the curve. The red circle shows where to place the rolled up towel.

10. Perform regular vigorous exercise

Performing activity that gets your heart racing for for 20 to 30 minutes, three to four times a week, is a minimum level of physical activity that the human body is designed to undertake for its own maintenance. Exercise reduces stress chemicals that can amplify pain.

A study of over 100 women with long-term neck pain looked at various stretches and exercises to alleviate neck pain. The study found no difference in the effectiveness of the various neck exercise regimes. The authors then examined pain scores in participants who performed intense regular physical exercise. They found that 33% of the participants exercised three to four times a week vigorously and, that when compared to the rest of the group, those participants experienced a third less neck pain.

Sometimes it is difficult to advise exactly which physical exercise is the best to perform, as people have different causes for their neck pain. Trial and error is the best approach. Performing exercise that does not aggravate your pain is important. There may also be a limit to how long you can perform an activity without developing neck pain. It may be five minutes or even an hour. Often, if an activity is causing pain, it is causing pressure on a damaged structure or stretching a painful muscle.

Swimming often aggravates pain as you need to turn your neck when swimming. One patient solved this problem by wearing a snorkelling device when swimming, allowing them to breathe with their neck straight. Cycling, especially on a road bike, can also aggravate neck pain due to constant flexion of the neck when riding.

As discussed in Chapter 9, exercise depletes stress chemicals and leaves us feeling relaxed. Only exercise that raises our heart rate depletes stress chemicals, and this does not include walking. While walking can be enjoyed for recreation, for most people it is better to pursue more vigorous exercise.

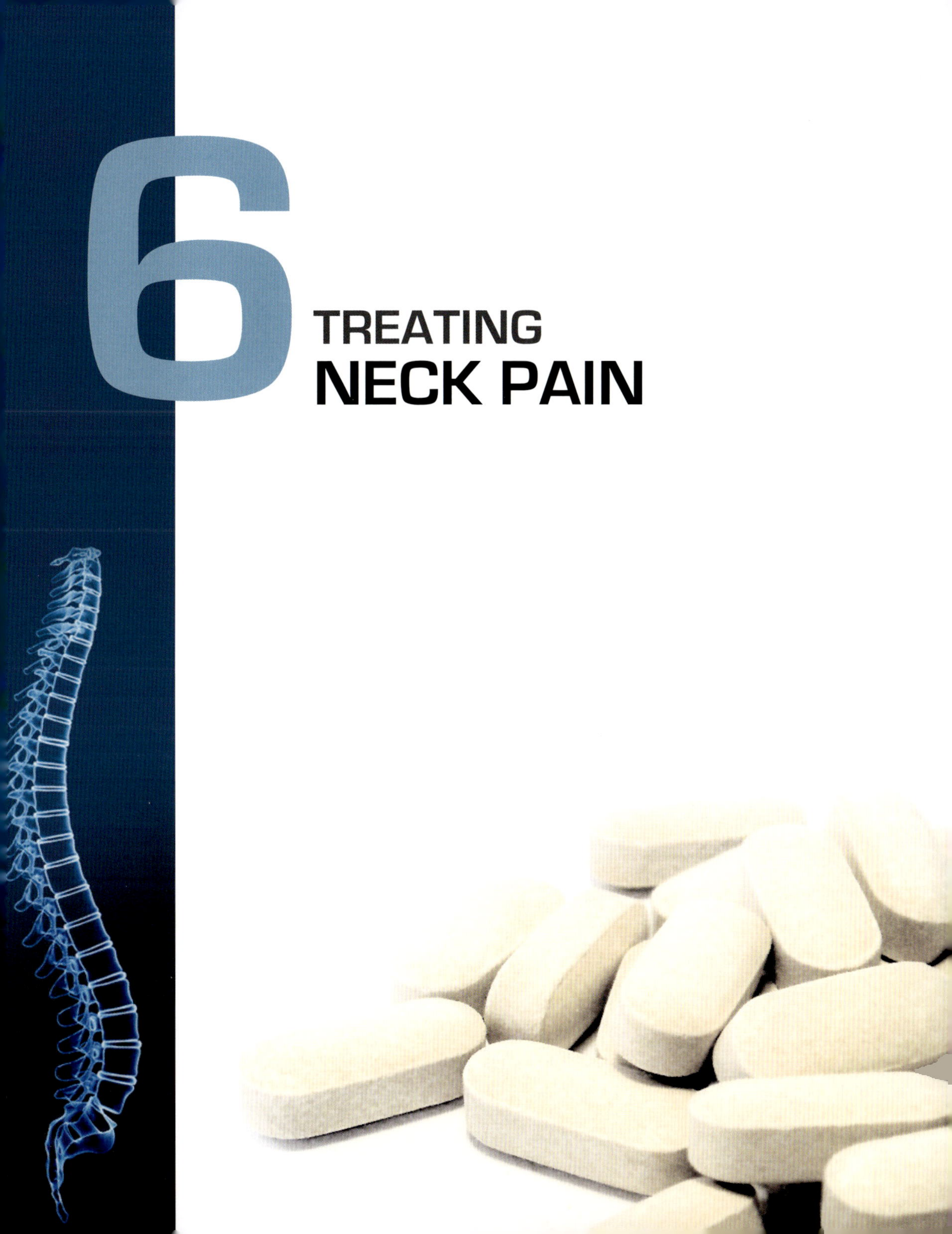

6 TREATING NECK PAIN

What do you do if your neck pain is not improving? There are many treatments available for neck pain and countless promises of miracle cures.

This chapter will outline some of the pharmaceutical options and commonly available hands-on treatments for neck pain. In clinical trials of painkillers, different medications are tested against chalk tablets (placebo) to see if they yield better results. Most vitamins, minerals and natural therapies are not tested to see if they are better than placebo, making them less-tested remedies.

What does the research show about the effectiveness of different treatment approaches? Clinical trials of neck pain have shown beneficial reductions in pain from manual therapies and acupuncture but these treatments do not usually eliminate pain altogether. A pragmatic approach is to start with simple treatments and progress to more invasive and therefore risky management options. It is also useful if the therapy can be performed at home, saving the time and money involved in travelling to appointments, taking time off work and paying health professionals' fees.

The disc is the most likely source of pain in the neck, and hence treatment aimed at the disc is best tried first. Pressure on the disc can increase pain, so it follows that reducing pressure can help alleviate pain. Simple traction exercises, such as lying with your head over the edge of the bed, and traction devices, as discussed in Chapter 5, are a good place to start in reducing neck pain. Traction reduces disc pressure and relaxes the surrounding muscles. The majority of patients using this approach have noticed a marked improvement in their symptoms, often over four to six weeks. Furthermore traction is very affordable, as it can be performed in your own home and without equipment.

Once traction has been performed, it is worth trying various treatment options for the tender muscles and tight joints. If there is improvement, then stick with the provider, otherwise change to another treatment approach. Pressure on the disc also causes muscle spasm and knots to form in the muscles surrounding the neck and head region. In turn the joints in the neck also can become stiff.

Some treatments are aimed at the muscle, such as massage, acupuncture or stretching. Others, like mobilisation or manipulation, are directed at the neck joints. Sometimes pain may improve for a short period only to return later. Often the painful muscle or tight joint is not the source of the pain but an underlying disc is the source, spreading pain into the muscles, causing joint tightness.

Medications

As described in Chapter 2, pain occurs due to electrical signals travelling via nerves to the brain. On the whole, medications that relieve pain do so by targeting the brain to reduce electricity and hence diminish pain, as shown in Figure 6.1. Medications do not generally act at the site of pain. In the case of the neck discs, the electrical spark produced is in response to pressure. Controlling pain by altering the pressure on the discs, through traction and changing the way you perform activity, is generally the best approach. However, medications may help when pain is severe or when you are waiting for improvement from treatment.

Medications can be divided into analgesics (painkillers) that are taken for pain (paracetamol, non-steroidal anti-inflammatories and opiates) and tablets that are taken regularly to reduce the brain's sensitivity to pain (anti-depressants, anti-epileptics, sedatives and anti-psychotics).

Medications are not always specific for the pain centres in the brain and may act on other parts of the brain to cause nausea, vomiting, fatigue and sleepiness, among other side effects.It is important to remember that there is no one tablet for all. Individuals often respond differently to different tablets, so what helps one person may not help another. Furthermore, one person may develop side effects while another develops no side effects. It is a case of trial and error most of the time, so if a tablet is not helping or causing side effects, you should go back to your doctor and try another one.

The analgesic medications commonly prescribed for neck pain are paracetamol, anti-inflammatories, opiates and tramadol. Combinations of medications are also commonly prescribed or can be purchased over the counter.

Paracetamol works on the brain pain pathways and is the first-line painkiller for muscle and joint pain due to its minimal side effects. The standard paracetamol tablet gives pain relief for approximately four hours. The main side effect of paracetamol is liver toxicity when given in overdose.

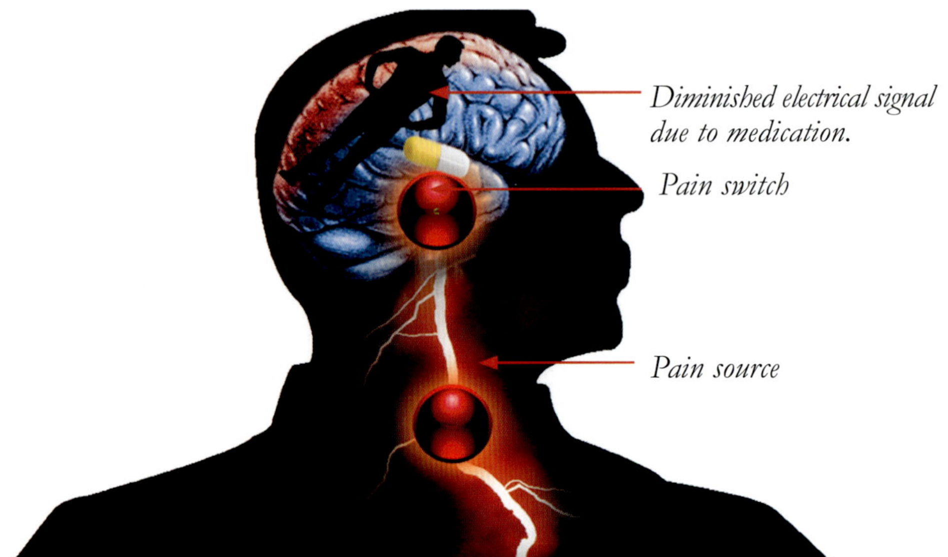

Figure 6.1
Medications reduce the electricity that conducts pain in the brain rather than act at the source of the pain.

Non-steroidal anti-inflammatory drugs include aspirin, ibuprofen, diclofenac, naproxen, meloxicam, and many others. In up to 15% of people taking these drugs, gastric bleeding occurs and can lead to stomach ulcers. If abdominal discomfort occurs, you should stop taking these tablets and see your doctor.

The consequence of gastric bleeding is often more severe in the elderly, and omeprazole (a tablet that reduces gastric acid) is often prescribed with a non-steroidal anti-inflammatory. These drugs can also increase asthma symptoms, so care needs to be taken when prescribing to asthmatics. Toxicity can also develop in the kidney and liver, usually with long-term usage. If taken intermittently, the incidence of side effects and toxicity is likely to be reduced when compared to taking tablets on a daily basis.

The commonly prescribed opiate medications are codeine, morphine, pethidine and methadone. Tramadol is an opiate-like medication. Codeine is usually the first-line opiate medication, but while it is effective for most people, 10% of the population cannot turn it into its active ingredient once swallowed. It is available over the counter combined with both paracetamol and ibuprofen. Taken in these combinations, it is thought to be slightly more effective. Codeine can cause drowsiness, which may be helpful at night if sleep is disturbed. Constipation is often the biggest problem if codeine is taken regularly. Stronger opiates including pethidine and morphine are also available on prescription. All opiates and tramadol are addictive if taken regularly for prolonged periods. If they are taken long term, patients often need to withdraw gradually rather than stop taking them abruptly.

Benzodiazepines are a group of medicines most widely prescribed for insomnia. Examples inclide diazepam, temazepam and clonazepam. Diazepam is better known as Valium and is a highly-addictive sleeping tablet. This group of tablets is sometimes prescribed to improve sleep and sometimes to reduce muscle spasm.

Baclofen and Orphenadrine, antihistamines often found in cold medications, are also prescribed for muscle spasm. Certain anti-depressants such as amitriptyline and nortriptyline are prescribed in low doses for neck pain. They are useful to help the patient sleep and may dull the pain a little as well. These tablets act on many receptors and have many side effects. Unfortunately, the elderly can experience dizziness, dry mouth and daytime sedation from these tablets. Anti-psychotics can also be prescribed in low doses to reduce pain by improving sleep.

Many medications used for epilepsy to reduce electricity in the brain are used for chronic pain. These include gabapentin, carbamazepine, pregabalin, and sodium valproate among many others.

Medications for neck pain are a useful addition to pain management but are best used for acute bouts of severe pain rather than used regularly. Many medications lose their effectiveness when taken regularly, as the brain becomes familiar with the medication and responds less. This tolerance leads to patients requiring escalating doses of medications to achieve the same effect. This is especially true for opiates.

Manual Therapy

Manual therapy is any therapy that is performed by hand. For neck pain, this usually includes massage, mobilisation and manipulation. People with neck pain experience secondary muscle spasm and joint tightness. A cycle often develops where a deeper structure is damaged, such as the disc, which in turn creates muscle spasm and subsequent joint tightness, leaving the individual with a feeling of stiffness. A combination of treating the muscles together with mobilisation or manipulation of the joints may relieve the feeling of tightness.

Massage

Massage therapy can be gentle for relaxation or rigorous and stimulate pain. Massage therapy often heats the area and increases blood flow. There is also a feedback mechanism to the pain centres of the muscle, spinal cord and brain when the skin is massaged. People find massage useful for relief of symptoms. If pain is caused by muscles, then massage has the potential to relieve pain totally, such as for a muscle strain. However, if the pain is stemming from a deeper structure such as the disc, joint or bone, massage may offer short-term alleviation but is unlikely to resolve the problem long term.

When a person has experienced pain for several months or longer, muscle knots are often widespread. Muscle knots develop in the muscles of the front of the neck, back of the neck and the shoulder muscles. The tight muscles do not work as they are designed, as they are shorter when contracted. Contracted muscles will in turn create changes in how joints move, often creating increased pressure on joints.When treating muscle knots, deep tissue massage or sports massage is often required. This applies more pressure on the muscle and can often result in pain, sometimes for several days after the treatment. This is a normal response to deep-tissue massage, and after several treatment sessions, the post-treatment pain often eases as the knots reduce in size.

Mobilisation

Mobilisation is like manipulation (cracking of the joints) but is performed with less vigour and no sudden forces. The joint is slowly moved and stretched. It is gentler than manipulation and achieves similar results. Therapists are often trained to both mobilise and manipulate joints, and choose which technique to use on a case-by-case basis.

Manipulation

Manipulation of joints is a sudden, vigorous movement used classically by chiropractors to improve spinal pain. It is an ancient art of healing, and many people swear by its effectiveness to relieve symptoms in their neck and back. While manipulation may give short-term relief, it is rarely long-lasting and often requires repeat visits, as it is not directed at the cause of pain. Figure 6.2 shows a therapist performing manipulation of the neck.

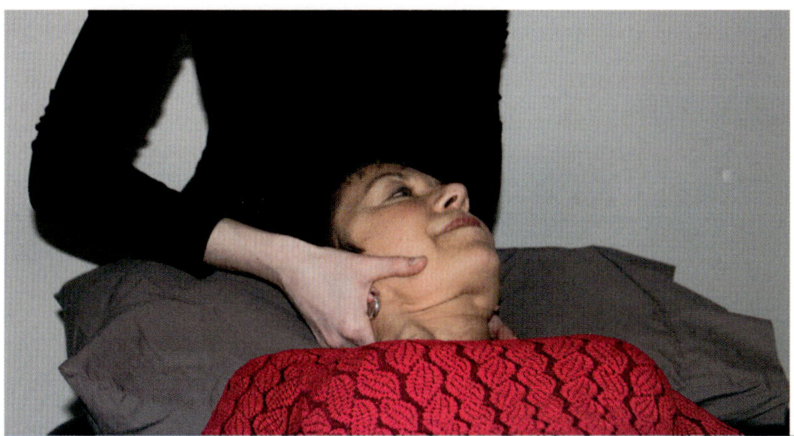

Figure 6.2
Manipulation of the neck.

Dry needling/Acupuncture

In acupuncture a thin needle is inserted into soft tissues such as the skin, muscle, tendon or ligament (Figure 6.3). The needle is often inserted into the muscle knot (an exquisitely tender region of the muscle) and produces a dull aching sensation. The needle irritates the muscle and after several sessions may relax the muscle knot. It is very safe and bleeding is often minimal, as the needle is small and cannot easily penetrate blood vessels.

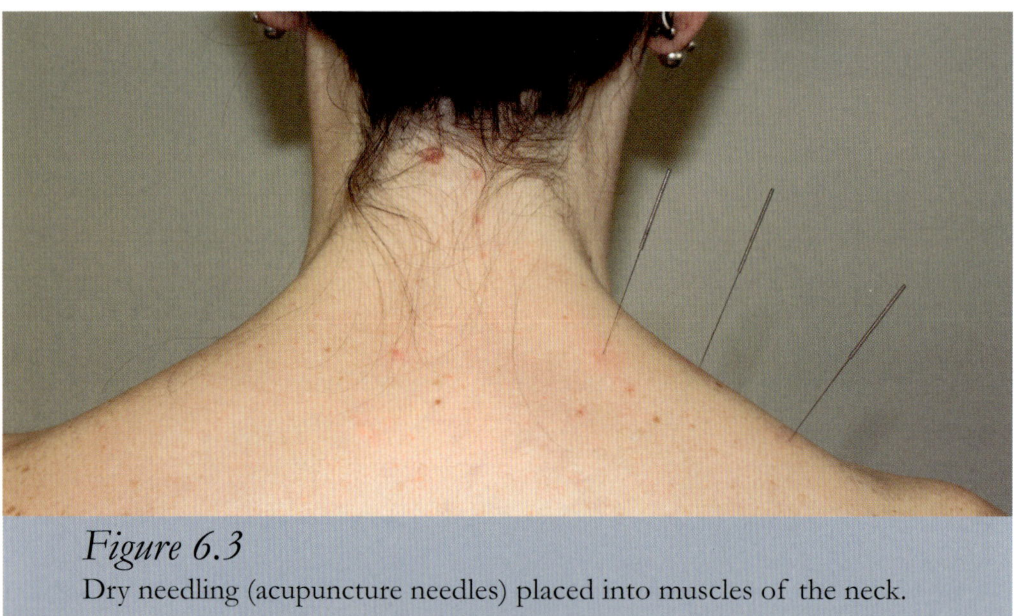

Figure 6.3
Dry needling (acupuncture needles) placed into muscles of the neck.

Injections

Several injection therapies have been promoted for low back and neck pain, including Botox, prolotherapy (injecting an irritant to stimulate healing), salt water (saline) and anaesthetic injections. In studies of low back pain, headache and migraine, saline injections have been found to be just as effective as prolotherapy and Botox.

When a large well-conducted study[13] showed that prolotherapy and saline injections gave similar improvements for low back pain, I started injecting saline into muscle knots because it is cheap, effective and has minimal side effects.

In 2006, I treated 100 consecutive patients with long-term low back pain (pain present for an average of six years) with saline injections[14]. I injected both the back muscles and ligaments with saline. In over a third of the patients the pain completely resolved and many others improved. I have used saline injections for over 10 years, with good relief of muscle pain for those suffering from neck pain, when treatments such as physiotherapy, chiropractic, osteopathy and exercises have not helped.

Over the past two years I have trained in ultrasound guided procedures: injections into muscle under ultrasound show stretching of the fibres as saline spreads into the muscle. Injections of solution are likely to reduce muscle knots by directly forcing muscle fibres apart.

A disc prolapse in the neck can irritate a nerve and cause sharp shooting pain, pins and needles, and numbness in the arm and hand. Steroids can be injected around the nerve to improve these symptoms. Injections are called transforaminal epidural injections or interlaminar epidural steroid injections and are often performed under guidance by CT Scan or X-ray to ensure correct placement and minimise side effects.

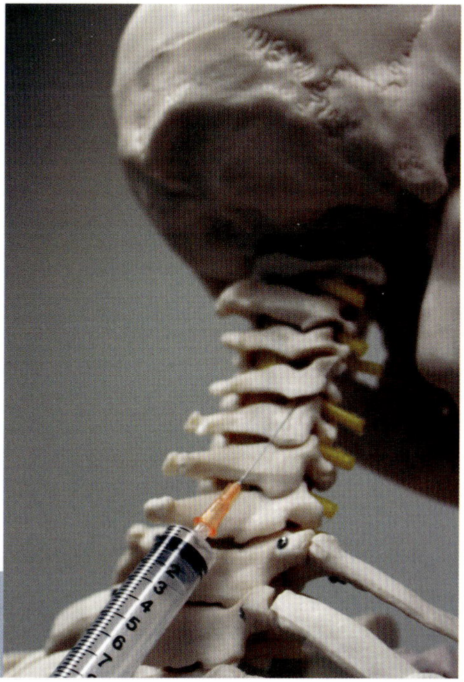

Figure 6.4
Injection of a facet joint.

The facet joints may also be injected with steroids under X-ray or ultrasound (Figure 6.4). Another treatment for the facet joints is to destroy the nerves that supply the joint, therefore stopping any electricity conducting pain to the brain. The nerve may regrow but the procedure may provide 12 or more months pain relief.

Surgery for neck pain

Sometimes neck pain does not respond to conservative management and surgery is considered. If severe neck pain is ruining someone's life and their scan shows a problem amenable to surgery, the most common operations are discectomy, fusion, disc replacement, foraminotomy and laminectomy.

Discectomy

Discectomy is the removal of part of the disc that has squeezed out of the disc wall (Figure 6.5). Usually the disc will shrink with time, but sometimes the disc prolapse persists and continues to compress the nerve that supplies the arm. Traction therapy has been shown to reduce the operation rate in disc prolapse and is therefore worth trying prior to considering discectomy. Return to work after a discectomy often depends on the type of job the person does. Desk-bound workers return to work quicker than those who perform heavy manual work.

The operation takes approximately one hour and patients are out of bed and often walking to the toilet on the day of their surgery. Patients usually return home within a few days. Complications can include a recurrent disc protrusion where some more material squeezes out of the disc. This occurs in 2–3% of people in the first year, and up to 10% of people in the first 10 years after surgery.

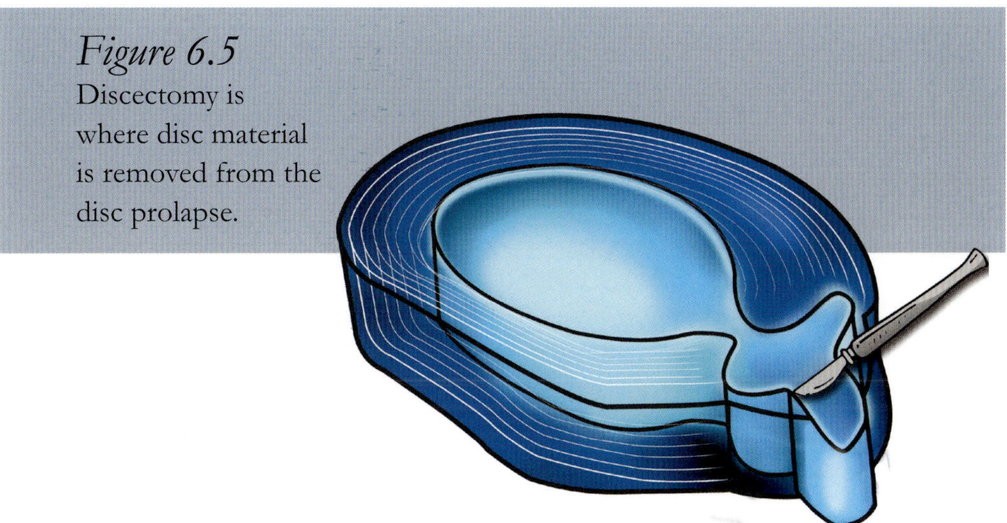

Figure 6.5
Discectomy is where disc material is removed from the disc prolapse.

Fusion

In patients where the disc has narrowed and lost the ability to absorb pressure, a fusion can be performed. This is a procedure where the bones are fixed together with screws (Figure 6.6), plates or even a cage so that they move as one unit and pressure is eased off the disc. A few days' bed rest is required after the operation, and patients usually go home within a week. One percent of patients can get post-operative infections and in up to 5% of patients the vertebrae do not fuse.

In a healthy spine all the discs absorb some pressure and allow some movement. However, if one level is fused it can no longer absorb pressure, and extra movement and pressure can occur in the discs surrounding the fusion. This can eventually lead to damage of surrounding discs, which may require further levels in the spine to be surgically fused. The extra pressure can also lead to pain arising from adjacent discs. This is especially true if the spine is subject to significant physical loads or trauma such as whiplash injuries.

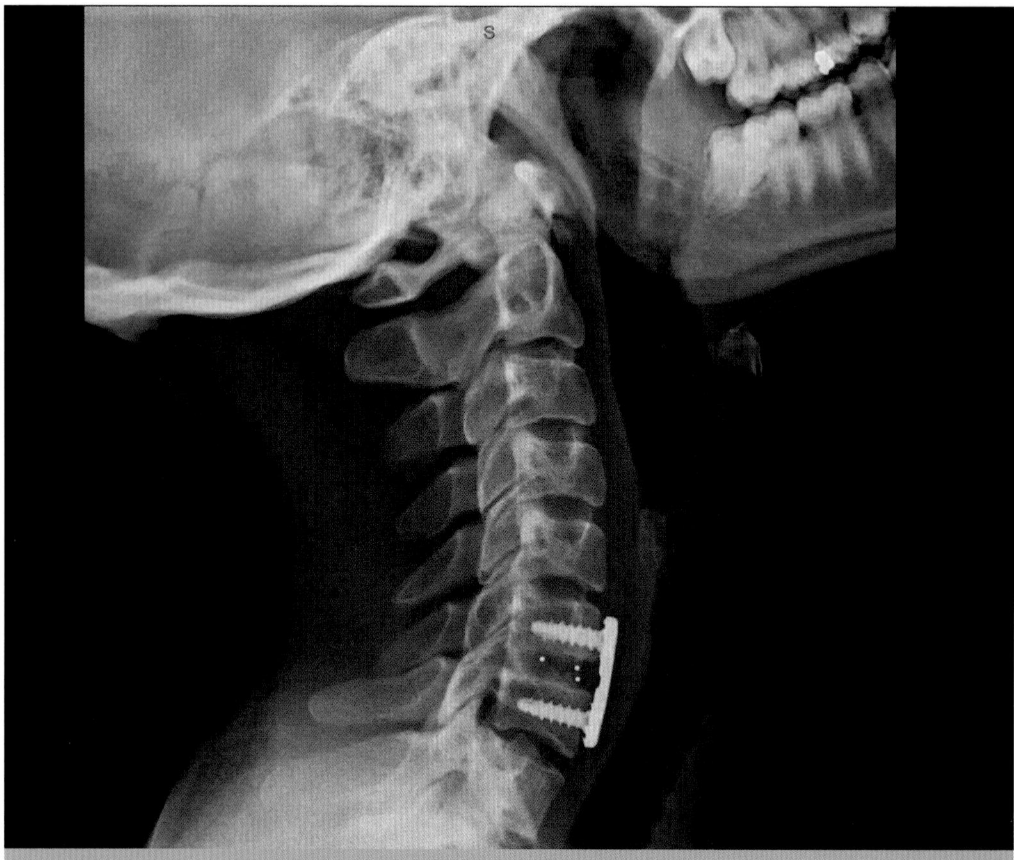

Figure 6.6
This X-ray shows a single level fusion between the sixth and seventh vertebrae of the neck.

If you have a fusion of the spine and continue to maintain postures that place increased pressure on the discs or have accidents, you risk damaging the discs at the level above or below the fusion. It is not true that the spine is as good as a new one once a fusion has been performed.

In fact, it is prudent to reduce forces on the spine after a fusion.

In a follow-up study after discectomy and fusion of the neck, nearly 75% of patients developed adjacent disc-level deterioration. Twenty percent of the study group had a further operation, most commonly to fuse the adjacent level disc that had deteriorated. On the whole, around two-thirds of patients have good relief of symptoms with a cervical spine discectomy and/or fusion in the first 10 years. As time progresses, however, the likelihood of adjacent disc deterioration increases, as people are more likely to experience falls or motor-vehicle accidents as time progresses. The accumulation of pressure over time may also compress the discs surrounding a fusion.

A study compared one group of people who had a disc fusion in the neck and another group of people without fusion of the neck. MRI scans were compared for both groups 10 years apart. The group with the fusion had accelerated adjacent disc changes such as dehydration, narrowing and reduction of space where the nerves exit from the neck[15].

An MRI scan is the best way to evaluate whether discs have normal structure and hydration. When evaluating a patient for a fusion operation at one level of the neck, it is essential to check the discs surrounding the proposed fusion. If one level is fused then extra pressure is placed on the surrounding discs. If the surrounding discs have good structure and hydration, they may be able to absorb pressure for decades. However, if the discs adjacent to the fusion are damaged (annular tear, dehydrated, narrowed, bulging or prolapsed), they will not be able to absorb the extra pressure in the years and decades following a fusion.

Both the state of the adjacent discs and the age of the patient are important when making decisions on fusion of the neck. A patient who is over 60 may live a further 20 years and is less likely to engage in sports or other activity placing them at risk of trauma. On the other hand, someone aged 20 may live for another 60 years. There is ample time for trauma such as motor-vehicle accidents, falls and sporting accidents that place the adjacent discs at risk of damage. Fusion of the neck needs a thorough assessment before being carried out, as the person should be concerned about the next few decades and not only the next few months.

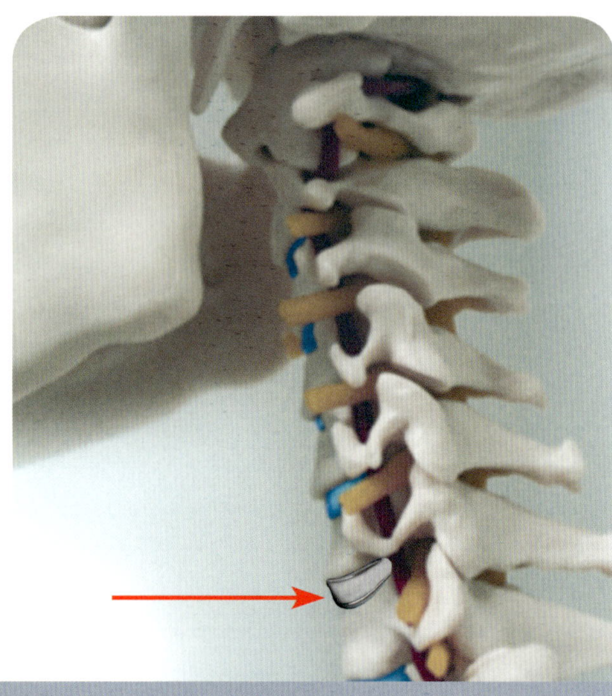

Figure 6.7
The disc has been removed and replaced by an artificial disc.

Disc replacement

Disc replacement has been developed as an alternative to spinal fusion. The damaged disc is replaced with an artificial disc designed to allow some movement in the spinal segment rather than stop movement altogether. This is a relatively new procedure, although it has been used in Europe for more than 15 years and has recently been approved in the United States. It is still considered experimental compared with spinal fusion. Figure 6.7 shows a disc replacement between two vertebrae. It is prudent to exhaust all conservative measures prior to considering disc replacement as it is still relatively new and its long-term results are uncertain.

CASE STUDY: *Jacqui*

Jacqui had an accident four years ago when her nephew stumbled onto her while she was lying on the ground. A few years later her pain worsened while at the gym. She had two years of physiotherapy and then sought advice from a surgeon. A scan showed a disc protruding at C6/7 (Figure 6.8) and she had a fusion operation in 2013 (Figure 6.9). A few months later her pain returned. A new scan (Figure 6.10) showed the disc above the fusion prolapsed. Further surgery such as discectomy/fusion or disc replacement was contemplated.

Jacqui started treatment including traction and postural advice to reduce the pressure on her lower neck. Within a few weeks she was pain free. She still has good disc heights and is likely to avoid a further operation to her neck.

If disc problems are present, adequate pain management, including traction, should be tried before contemplating any surgical procedure.

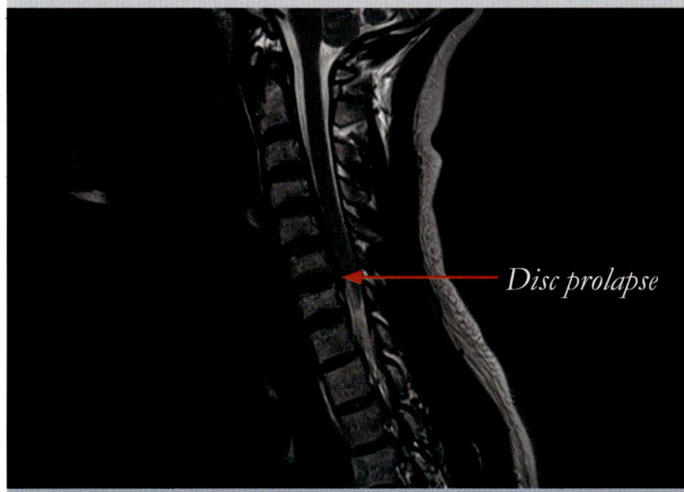

Figure 6.8
The disc between the sixth and seventh vertebrae is protruding.

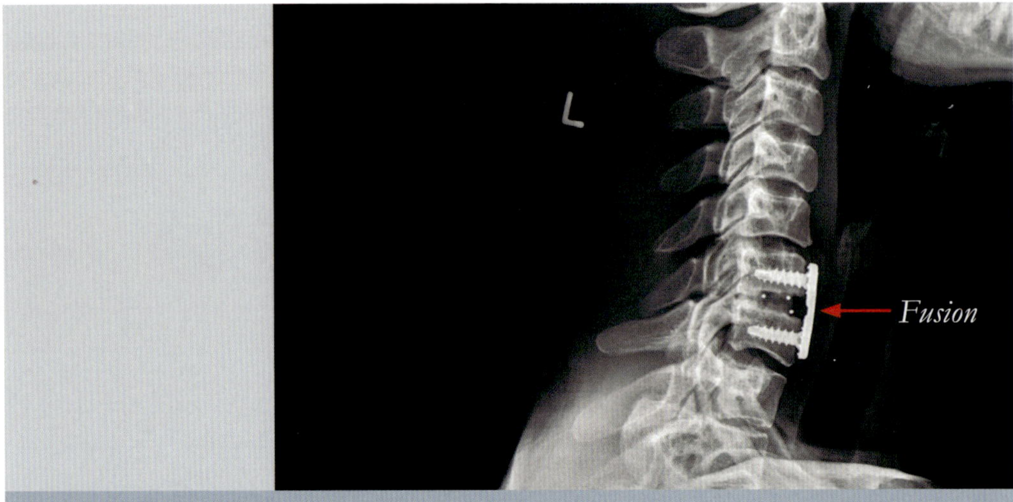

Figure 6.9
An X-ray shows a fusion performed with metal plate and screws between the sixth and seventh vertebrae.

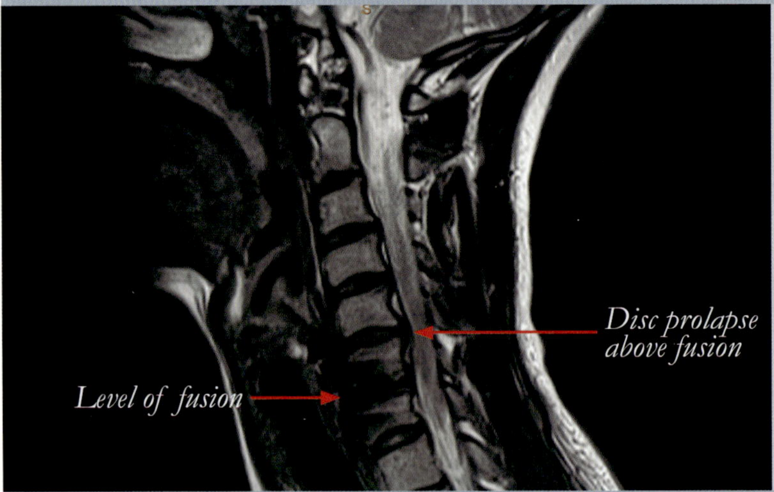

Figure 6.10
The metal device used in the fusion shows as a blurred area and the disc above the fusion protrudes near the spinal cord.

Foraminotomy

The nerves that exit the spinal cord at the neck travel through a passage called a foramen (opening). This opening can become encroached by structures such as the disc (disc prolapse), bones (burrs and spurs from bones) and ligaments. Once this happens, nerves can be irritated as they exit and produce symptoms down the arms such as sharp shooting pain, pins and needles, numbness and tingling.

A foraminotomy is an operation where structures that encroach on the opening are surgically removed to increase the opening so the nerve does not become compressed or irritated.

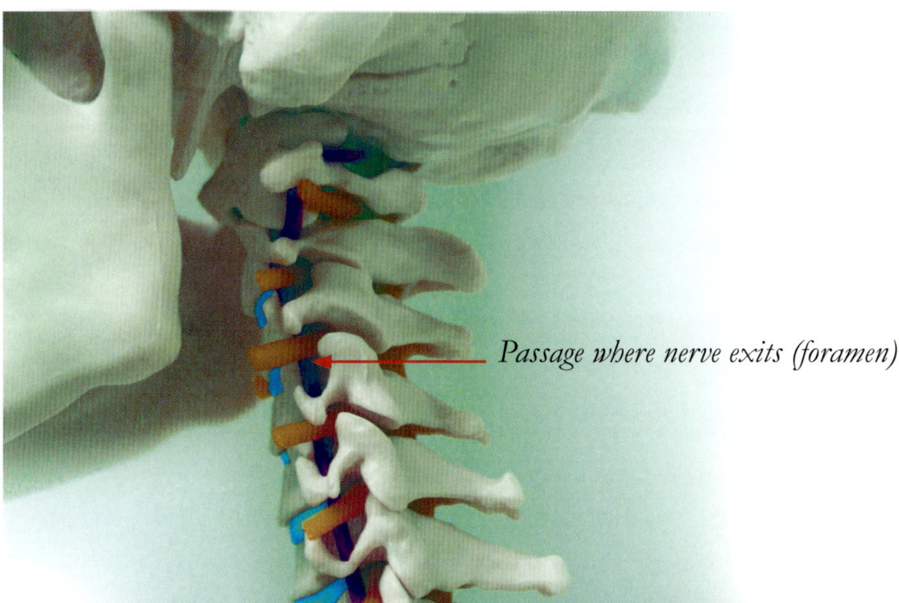

Figure 6.11
The passage (foramen) in the neck through which the nerves travel to the arms and hand.

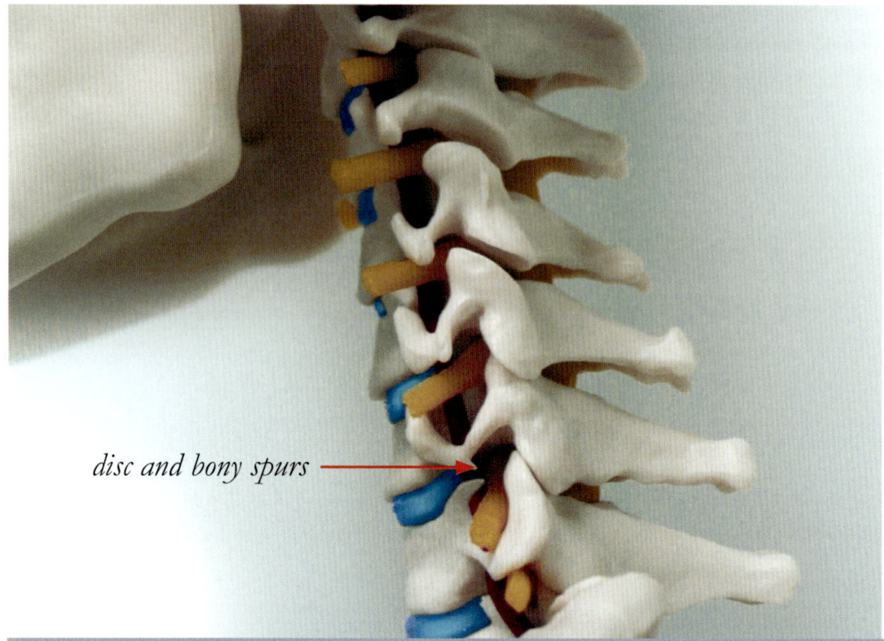

Figure 6.12
Disc and bony spurs protrude backwards to reduce the size of the opening where the nerve exits. This can often create pins and needles down to the fingers on certain movements of the neck or at night when asleep.

CASE STUDY: *Sally*

Approximately 25 years ago, Sally fell, hit her chin on the ground and developed jaw and neck pain. Over the years pain spread into the head and down both arms. Sometimes the pain was sharp and shooting, and she had tried several medications. When she was seen in 2012 she was taking medicines including methadone, gabapentin, tramadol and Sevredol. She was taking more than 20 analgesic tablets a day when she presented.

Her MRI scan (Figure 6.13), showed marked disc narrowing at C5/6. The CT scan (Figure 6.14) of the neck, which gives excellent bone detail, showed the bone spurs which develop in response to increased pressure falling on the bone (the pressure that is no longer absorbed by the faulty disc).

The bony spurs were causing nerve pressure, creating symptoms down into the arms, including sharp, shooting pain, pins and needles and numbness and tingling. Sally had a foraminotomy in 2014 that relieved the symptoms down the arm and hand.

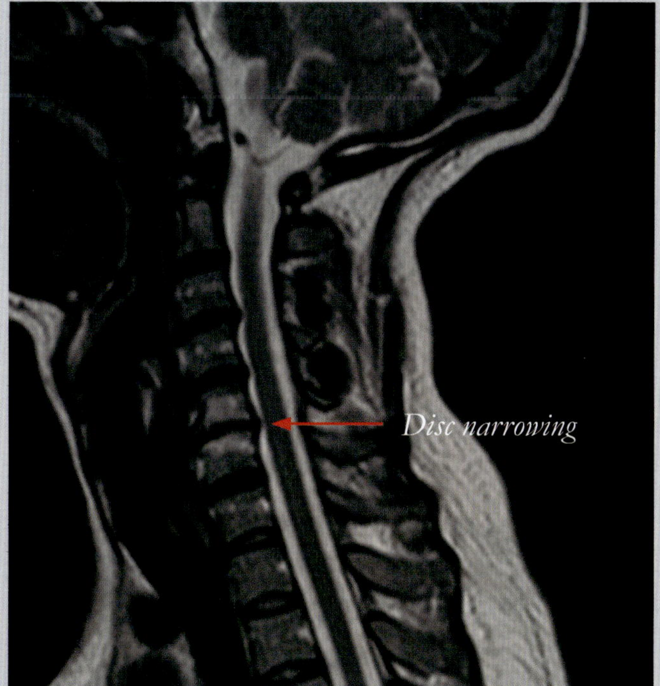

Figure 6.13
The MRI scan shows disc narrowing between the fifth and sixth vertebrae in the neck. There are also bone spurs which are contributing to the narrowing of the opening where the nerves exit.

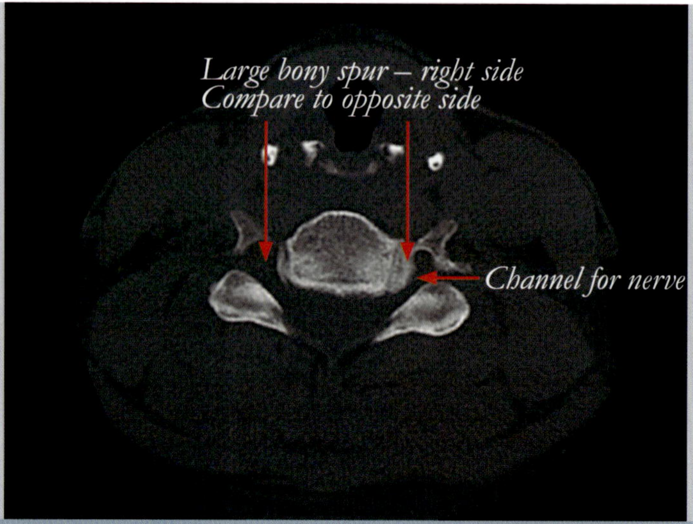

Figure 6.14
The CT scan shows a cross-section of the neck with good bone detail. On the right hand side a bone spur (osteophyte) is seen protruding into the channel where the nerve exits the neck to travel into the arm and hand.

Laminectomy

A laminectomy is a surgical procedure to relieve pressure on the spinal cord. Disc, ligament and bone spurs (osteophytes) can protrude backwards into the spinal cord and reduce the space around the spinal cord (called spinal stenosis). Lamina refers to the bony covering at the back of the spinal column. In a laminectomy, a small section of bone covering the back of the spinal cord is removed to make room for the spinal cord which then has room to float backwards.

Once pressure falls on the spinal cord there can be disruption of nerves which travel within the spinal cord (myelopathy) from the brain to the whole body. Myelopathy can produce problems with the bowel and bladder, disruptions in the way you walk, and make it difficult to carry out fine motor skills with the hands such as doing up buttons. The bony spurs are a result of excess pressure falling on the vertebrae and hence coexist with damaged discs in the neck. The bony spurs most commonly occur in the lower two levels of the neck (C5/6 and C6/7) as these two levels are where most of the force is transmitted from the head. To prevent bony spurs developing in the presence of disc damage, it is imperative to reduce pressure on the discs by maintaining good neck posture.

CASE STUDY: *Ashley*

Ashley, a 55 year old year old male, noticed tennis elbow symptoms in the left elbow after lifting an exercise machine in May 2014. The pain soon spread to the whole left arm. Initially he developed pins and needles and numbness in one hand followed by symptoms in both hands. He noticed his hands felt like cotton wool and fine movements such as doing up buttons felt different. He also started dropping cups of tea and other items.

Ashley went to see his local physiotherapist who diagnosed it was arising from his neck. He was then reviewed by a pain specialist who ordered an MRI scan of the neck. The MRI scan (Figure 6.15 and 6.16) showed narrowing of the discs at the lower neck and also extensive bony spurs which were best seen on a CT scan (Figure 6.17 and 6.18).

Ashley worked as a software developer with countless hours working on computers and laptops over many decades. Laptops with the flexed neck posture place significant pressure on the lower neck discs, causing narrowing over decades.

Surgery (laminectomy and foraminotomy) was performed in March 2015 to make space for the spinal cord and nerves that exit at the lower neck.

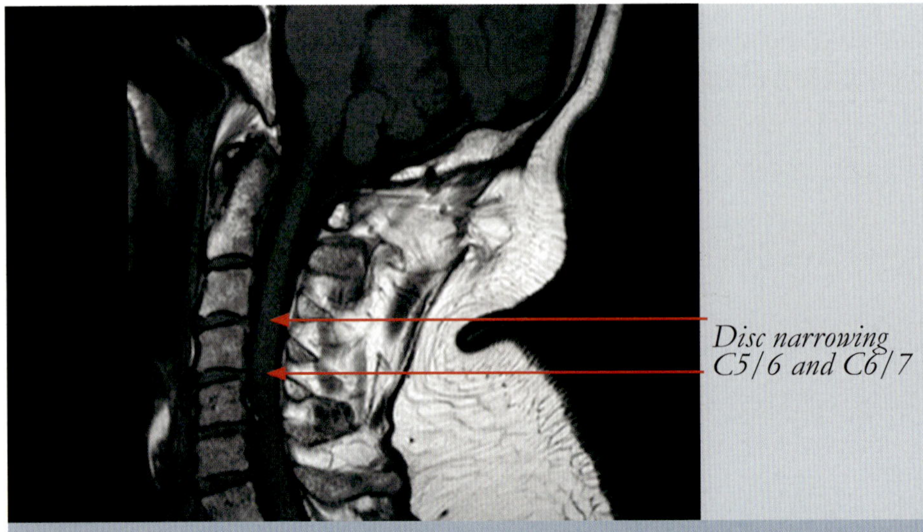

Figure 6.15
The MRI scan shows disc narrowing and protrusion at C5/6 and C6/7.

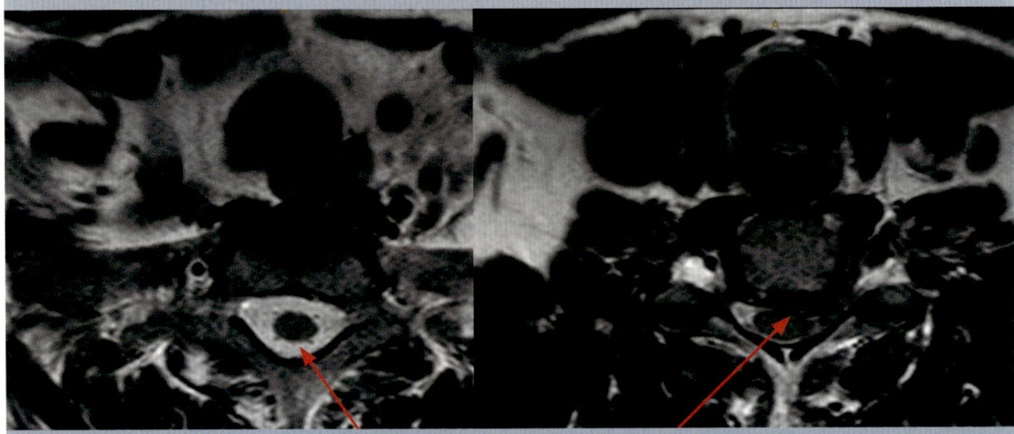

Figure 6.16
The arrow is pointing to the spinal column with the cord inside. The left-hand image from the C2/3 level shows spinal fluid (white) surrounding the cord while the right-hand image (C6/7) shows the disc has encroached on the space in front of the disc.

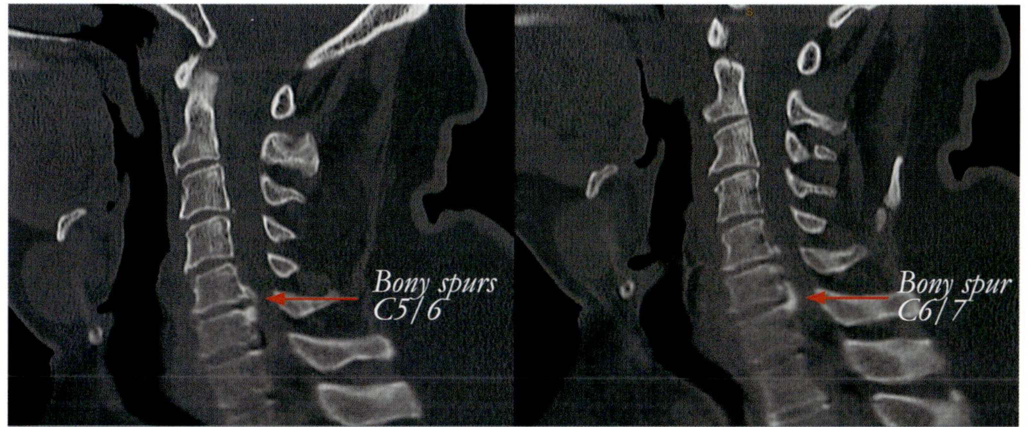

Figure 6.17

The above CT scans shows bony spurs better than MRI scans. The left-hand side shows bony spurs at C5/6 and the right-hand side shows these at C6/7.

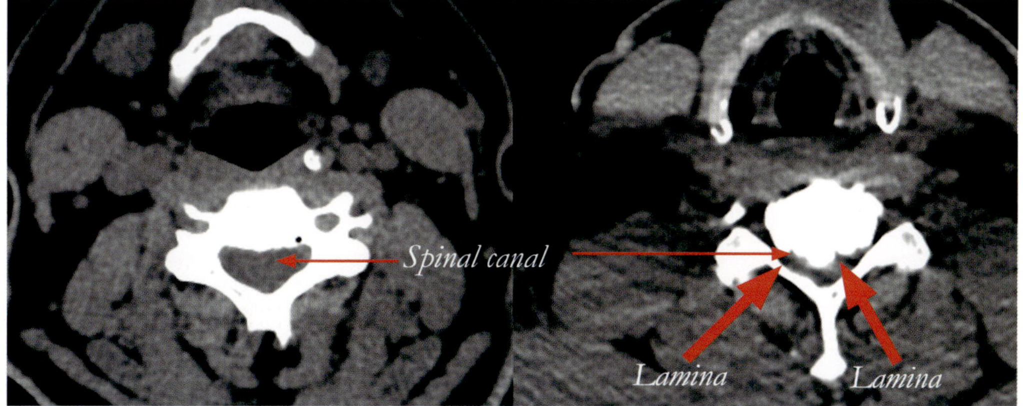

Figure 6.18

The above CT scans shows a cross-section of the neck. The left-hand side shows a normal shape spinal canal while the right shows bony spurs reducing the spinal canal. The thick red arrows point to the bone called the lamina which can be surgically removed to allow increased space for the spinal cord (laminectomy).

7

HEADACHE & MIGRAINE

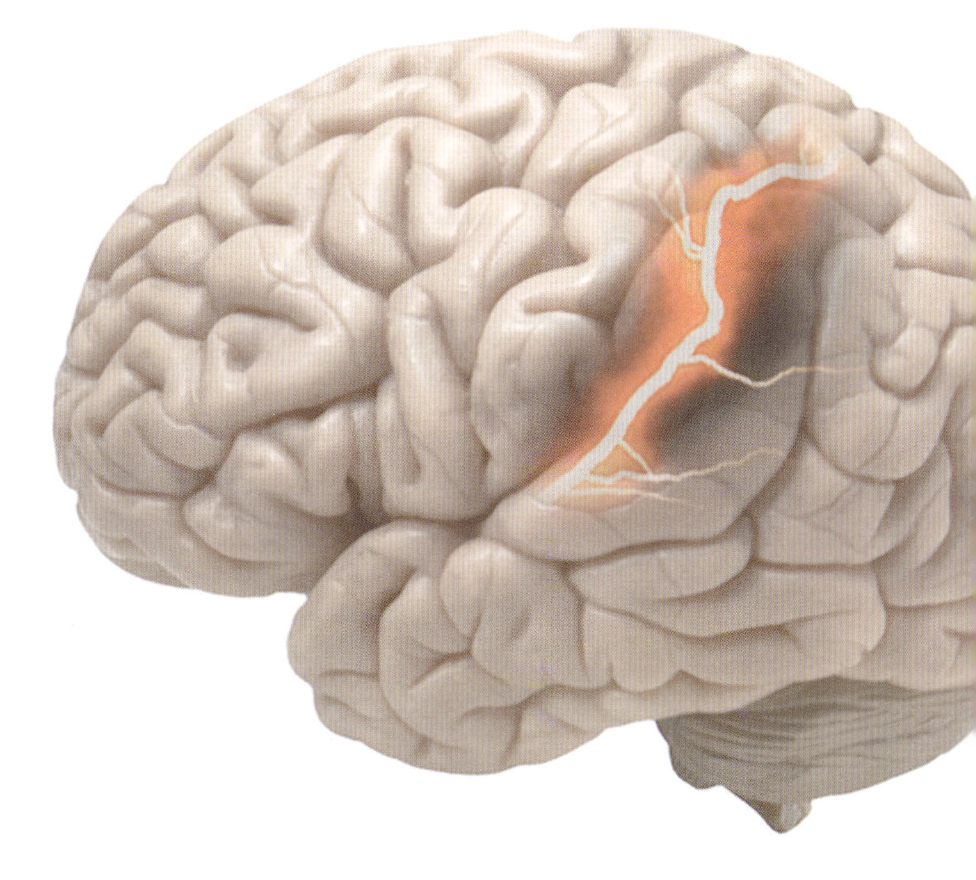

Headache disorders

Headache is the most common neurological problem in the world. Approximately 50% of the population regularly have headaches, and 14% have migraines. The cost of headache and migraine runs into billions of dollars worldwide every year. The occurrence of tension headache and migraine is three times more common in females and is highest between the ages of 25 and 55.

Headache is one of the oldest medical conditions affecting mankind, likely to have been around long before the written word. Migraine headache was first recorded during the Mesopotamian Era in about 3,000 B.C. A few notable migraine sufferers throughout history include Thomas Jefferson, Julius Caesar, Cervantes, Sigmund Freud, Ulysses S. Grant, Lewis Carroll and Vincent van Gogh.

The origin of headache disorders has been elusive, despite significant research. Headache and migraine has been mostly treated with trial-and-error approaches. Some of the treatments prescribed by early physicians such as Galen and Hippocrates included drilling a hole in the skull to free "evil spirits", purges and bloodletting, applying a hot iron to the site of pain, and inserting a clove of garlic through an incision in the temple.

Beta-blockers, the most effective migraine preventative medication, were discovered by accident in 1966. A patient was experiencing chest pain from the heart and was given a beta-blocker for the heart pain. He was simultaneously experiencing a migraine attack that subsided with the beta-blocker medication. Subsequent research has confirmed the usefulness of beta-blockers for migraine prophylaxis. Beta-blockers "block" signals from adrenaline and noradrenaline which are stress chemicals released in the brain and body. In my doctoral thesis, "The Adrenaline Model of Headache Causation" was formed and explained why beta-blockers helped people with headache disorders.

Migraine

The basic difference between migraine and headache is the intensity of symptoms. Both are charactherised by pain experienced in the head, but someone with migraine expereinces severe pain, often accompanied by associated symptoms of nausea, vomiting, light intolerance, sound intolererance and flashing lights (aura). Migraine is classified into two main categories: migraine without aura and migraine with aura.

Migraine is best defined as the hereditary predisposition for people to experience heightened sensations. People with migraine experience heightened sensations of light, sound, pain, touch and smell. The genetic difference is due to electrical channels in the brain that open up much more quickly, with greater amounts of electricity created in the brain. Greater amounts of electricity create increased pain and other sensations.

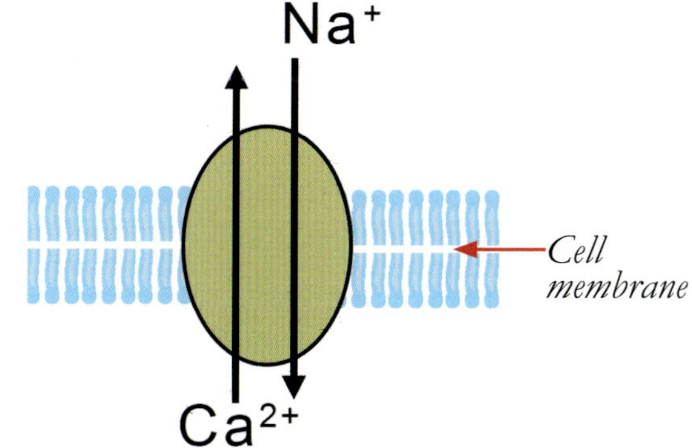

Figure 7.1
A sodium/calcium ion channel. Ion channels in the brain are different in people who experience migraine. They open more quickly and produce more electrical signals.

The visual aura represents spontaneous generation of electricity in the part of the brain that controls vision. Hence, when a person experiences an aura, they are experiencing a spontaneous electrical signal generated in the brain. People with migraine do not necessarily experience headache pain. Many migraine patients have experienced the aura such as flashing lights but no pain.

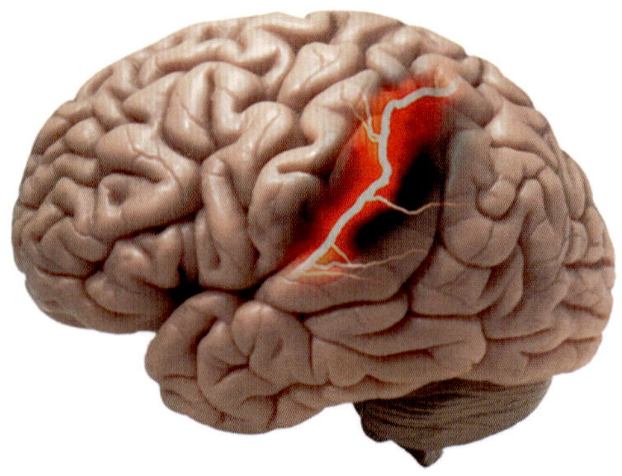

Figure 7.2
The aura represents electricity signals generated in the part of the brain that experiences sensations, mostly light and less often odour.

Epilepsy is another condition where spontaneous electricity can be created in the brain, but it occurs specifically in the centres for movement. This is why people with epilepsy experience movement of their arms and legs. Migraine can be thought of as epilepsy in the part of the brain that experiences sensations such as pain, light, sound and smell. The two conditions can co-exist in the same person, and if you have migraine you are three to four times more likely to experience epilepsy than someone without migraine. Conversely those who experience epilepsy are three to four times as likely to experience migraine. Medications that suppress electrical signals in the brain are used for both migraine and epilepsy.

As explained in Chapter 2, when the intensity of pain increases, pain sensations can spread. For people with migraine, pain is more likely to spread as they produce more electrical signals in their brains. Symptoms arising from the neck spread quickly into the head, causing headache. People who experience migraine are six times more likely to experience widespread body pain (fibromyalgia) and twice as likely to experience low back pain[16].

CASE STUDY: *Mark*

Mark presented in 2014 with headache and neck pain. He had experienced headache as well as migraine with aura for over 15 years. Five months before he presented, he had aggravated his headache and neck pain after plastering a ceiling for long periods. Below is an email he forwarded prior to his consultation.

Dr Kanji,

I am writing to you to request a consultation with you at your clinic. I am a 30yo male and have been suffering a sore neck and intense frontal headaches for the better part of 5 months. I have also experienced intense photo-phobia at times over the duration. The headaches are causing me the most trouble and have kept me from working since April. I am a gib stopper (plasterer) and painter. My symptoms started very suddenly whilst working overhead on a complex ceiling as part of an architecturally designed house. I have been to see a specialist who has conducted X-ray, and MRI scans. Unfortunately no one seems to be able to tell me what is going on or what is causing my symptoms.

I am starting to get desperate as I can't seem to find a local physician with relevant experience … Your extensive experience with this sort of thing leads me to think you might be able to offer me some useful advice.

I am concerned that I appear to have a disc bulge at C3/4 and that this is pushing on my occipital nerve and causing my symptoms. I personally believe there is evidence to support this theory in the MRI scan (I have a copy and have cross referenced this against many other "positive" MRI scans sourced from the internet and also from family members who have suffered similar injuries and have MRI scans confirming this). However when I raise this with either my gp or my specialist they just laugh and tell me the radiographer who read my scan was very experienced and there is no evidence to suggest there is anything wrong. I believe he may have missed something.

The specialist I have been seeing has requested a bone scan to look for any spurs etc that may have been missed on the MRI and X-rays. If my theories are indeed correct, then I feel this is unnecessary and I would rather not go through this procedure as I am concerned about the amount of radiation exposure and also the waste of money.

My headache presents as a near constant frontal dull ache situated above and behind both eyes. I also experience short term intense, stabbing, hot pain in the same areas that lasts anywhere between 10 seconds and 10 minutes. These pains are so severe that I am fully incapacitated and have to drop whatever I am doing. I am in agony. Often when these intense pains occur I lose my balance. Any prolonged activity with my neck in either a flexion or extension exacerbates these stabbing headaches for 24 to 48 hours. These symptoms are least active when I am lying down, and I am not usually aware of them until after getting up in the morning. Usually within moments of getting vertical, the headache comes on. Sometimes it can take a few minutes. As the MRI scan was done with me lying down, I am concerned that this may not have shown the full extent of any disc bulging/herniation.

My neck muscles are almost always in a state of spasm, despite having acupuncture, physio and more recently bowen therapy. All of which caused severe headache reaction despite helping to temporarily relax the muscles.

I am normally a fit, strong and very active young man and am starting to really struggle emotionally and psychologically due to the lack of any diagnosis, the constant debilitating pain and not being able to work or do many of the things I love.

I look forward to hearing from you.

Kind regards and thanks,

Mark

Mark had a small disc bulge in the cervical spine which I suspected was the cause of his symptoms. Although the disc bulge was small, this was probably a disc prolapse that had reduced in size since the time of his injury and the time of the scan (several months). Mark had a history of migraine with aura, which predisposes him to amplify pain from minor tissue damage in the body, explaining why a small disc bulge may cause significant symptoms, whereas someone without migraine with aura might experience no pain from the same pathology.

People with migraine with aura have electrical channels in the part of their brains that experience sensations (light, sound, touch, pain and smell) that open up more quickly and produce more electricity, resulting in increased pain. Another important factor is his occupation as a plasterer. With the head extended for long periods of time plastering the ceiling, he was placing significant loading on the discs of his neck. Pain is a consequence of damage to a disc, the pressure placed on the disc and the electricity generated in the spinal cord and brain. Although the disc damage was minor, the pressure placed on the disc was significant and prolonged, and Mark's brain had a high sensitivity to pain.

Following my diagnosis, and the treatments I recommended, Mark's condition improved significantly. A few weeks later his mother, a retired physiotherapist, sent me this email. My job can often seem thankless, but this kind of email gives me the inspiration to continue working with people suffering chronic pain.

Dear Dr. Kanji,

You recently saw my son, Mark and that consultation with you, gave my son his life back. He had explored every possibility he could think of up till he discovered you and his coping power, which despite impressing me as a mother and a physio that it had lasted as well he had, it was definitely running out.

When all manual therapies had exacerbated his symptoms and the orthopedic surgeon had said there was nothing wrong, it was a hard battle to keep on going. From my experience his symptoms were definitely in line with a bulging disc at C3/4 but when the orthopod denied that we were hamstrung.

Then Mark discovered your website and his face lost the 20 years of stress, this had all given him, when you so quickly confirmed the diagnosis. The program you have recommended is already having a pain relieving effect and we hear his very welcome chuckles resurface.

As his mother I want to thank you from the bottom of my heart, for your care and treatment you have and are giving Mark.

As a retired physio, I am very very grateful for the study you have pursued on pain and spinal problems. It was an area that often left me frustrated at the lack of real understanding and how so often the medicos would suggest either the patient was an undeserving malingerer or simply a nutcase.

I was intrigued to read how a person with a history of migraines, experiences spinal disturbances differently to those without. How I wish I had known more about all this when in my own practice. However, I know that many many health professionals will benefit from your study and sharings and again I thank you so very much for all your dedication in this field.

At this time in our society where so much treatment, diagnosis and care is determined by how much it will cost, to find a doctor such as yourself who is still devoted to the true meaning of medicine is simply wonderful.

Mark gave me the book you so generously gifted him to give me - thank you so much. It answered so many of my wonderings. I specially appreciated the illumination of the hormonal stresses that ongoing pain creates and the use of saunas for ridding the buildup of such stress hormones. I now understand so much better the physiological cause of the psychological depression that accompanies such.

For all the above, I thank you from the bottom of my heart and just pray the work you do will attract more of the medical profession to remember what caring for patients is truly about.

Bless you.
Astrid

I also received an email from Mark four weeks after the consultation.

Hi Dr Kanji,

It has been a little over a month since I saw you and as discussed I want to give you an update on my condition.

I have been religiously keeping up with your suggestions including traction, sauna multiple times a week, and using the soft collar for prevention of further injury. I have also been doing gentle exercise in the pool prior to sauna. I am definitely doing a lot better! I have only used pain relief 4-5 times in the last month which is a huge reduction. As long as I don't do anything to aggravate it, my headache is dramatically reduced from where it was a month ago with increasingly large periods with almost no pain at all. It is definitely still there but 95% of the time the pain is at a level that is tolerable without medication. Day by day, slowly it is improving. I am also feeling much better in myself, including better energy levels, clearer thinking and happier disposition. I have hope that one day in the not-too-distant future I will be totally pain free.

Thank you so much for all your help with all of this, you are a wonderful human being and Doctor and I am truly grateful for having had the opportunity to consult with you.

Thank you once again and I hope life is treating you well.

Kind regards,

Mark

Headache and migraine triggers

Many headache triggers are common to both tension headache and migraine A study of 1,750 migraine sufferers attending a headache clinic investigated migraine triggers and found the triggers to be stress (80%), hormones in women (65%), not eating (57%), weather (53%), sleep disturbance (50%), perfume or odour (44%), neck pain (38%), lights (38%), alcohol (38%), smoke (36%), sleeping late (32%), heat (30%), food (30%), exercise (22%) and sexual activity (5%)[17].

CASE STUDY: *Chloe*

Chloe, a 39 year old woman, slipped over on a mat and hit the back of her head against a cupboard handle 18 months before seeing me. After this incident, she noticed worsening headache and migraine as well as pain at the back of her left shoulder. The pain radiated down her left arm with pins and needles and numbness and tingling into her left hand.

The frequency of migraine attacks increased from less than once a month to two or three times a week. The pain had radiated into the back of the left eye and was associated with nausea, vomiting and sensitivity to light and sound. When she presented she was taking Panadol, tramadol, ibuprofen and several other headache medications. An MRI scan of her head showed no major problems. She could not sleep due to her pain, despite several medicines for both sleep and pain. The migraines were not responding to medication and she was attending the emergency department of the local hospital for pethidine injections two to three times a week.

An X-ray and MRI scan of her neck were performed. These showed narrowed discs in the lower neck. Her neck had also straightened with the loss of the normal curve. She started treatments for her neck with traction, altering postures to reduce pressure on the discs, and wearing a soft collar intermittently. She improved rapidly and returned to work within two weeks.

Her medication intake reduced and she no longer attended the emergency department for pethidine injections.

Chloe's case, where a neck injury starts the cycle of increased migraines or headaches, is a common one. This vicious cycle is often accompanied by poor sleep and constant pain.

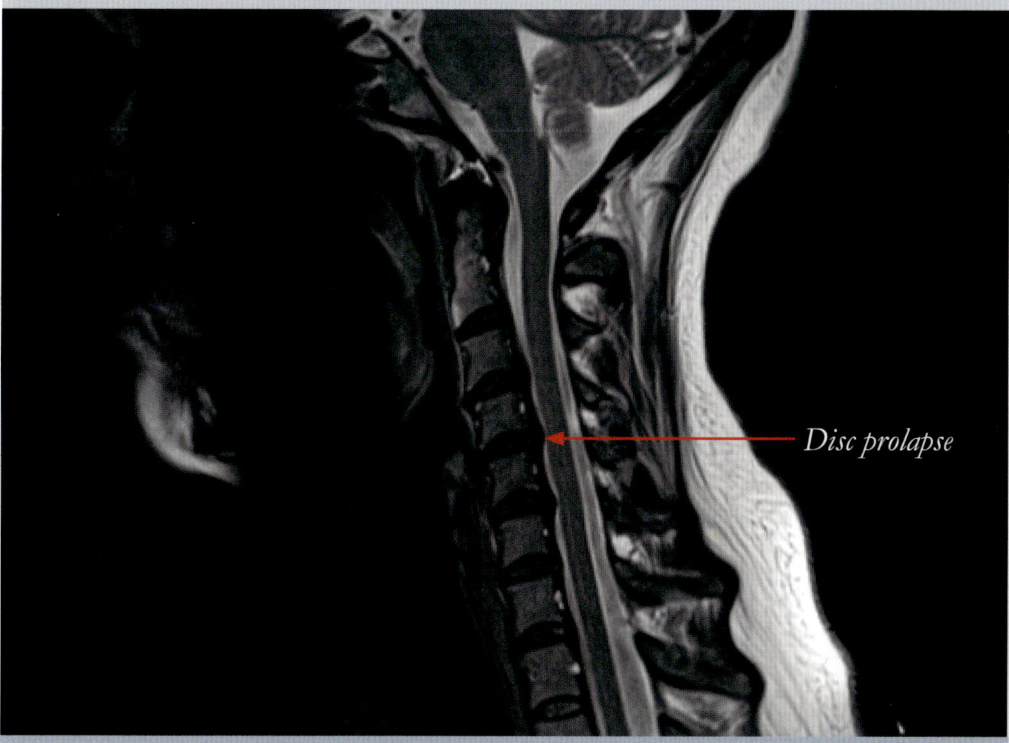

Figure 7.3
The MRI scan shows a straight neck as well as a disc prolapse between the fourth and fifth vertebrae in the neck.

Theories to explain headache

The most popular theory to explain headache pain used to be one based around dilated blood vessels. A specific heart medication (glyceryl tri-nitrate) is used for heart disease to dilate blood vessels. The spray also causes headache as a side effect leading to the mistaken belief that headache is due to blood vessel dilatation. Many health professionals still hold and publicise this belief, despite evidence to the contrary.

Dilated blood vessels are unlikely to cause headache for several reasons. First, glyceryl tri-nitrate causes delayed headache but the dilatation of blood vessels is immediate. Several tablets that dilate blood vessels are used to prevent migraine. Adrenaline can induce headache but constricts blood vessels rather than dilates them. One study showed no differences in blood flow in blood vessels when treating migraine attacks[18]. The most damning evidence is a study that performed MRI scans of the blood vessels when people were either experiencing migraine or were migraine free. There were no differences in the diameter of blood vessels among the two groups[19].

Glyceryl tri-nitrate causes headaches and has been used in headache trials to produce headaches and migraines. The mechanism of action is usually explained in terms of the vasodilatation caused by nitric oxide. Glyceryl tri-nitrate activates messengers that lead to the opening of electrical channels in the brain. The dilatation of blood vessels is coincidental rather than a cause of headache.

The Adrenaline Model of Headache Causation

The Adrenaline Model of Headache Causation was formed during my PhD, after I had examined volumes of research written about headache over the past 40 years. I examined the worldwide distribution of headache, headache triggers, headache medications, headache treatments and co-morbidities to develop a model that was consistent with what we knew about headache.

Signals generated from the body travel to the brain in small pockets of electricity. Once the electricity reaches the brain, pain centres experience where the pain is coming from and how severe the pain is, and other parts of the brain are activated, resulting in an emotional response. The Adrenaline Model of Headache Causation proposes that stress chemicals released in the brain and spinal cord attach to the electrical channels, opening them and ultimately increasing the electrical activity in the brain, resulting in increased pain. Chemicals released in the brain include adrenaline, noradrenaline, histamine and serotonin.

The Adrenaline Model of Headache Causation makes sense of many headache phenomena, including the fact that drugs that mimic adrenaline and adrenaline-producing tumours (phaechromocytoma) increase headache pain. The model explains why beta-blockers may be effective in reducing migraine, as beta-blockers block the activity of adrenaline. Adrenaline, noradrenaline, histamine and serotonin receptors are also the targets of many headache medications. Medications causing headache act on receptors that increase electricity in the pain pathways, and medications that help with headache reduce electricity in the pain pathways.

The distribution of headache and migraine throughout the world is also explained by the model. Migraine and headache are more common in colder European climates compared to Africa and Asia. Heat reduces the activity of the stress nervous system, so people experience less pain in the heat. They also feel more relaxed in a tropical climate. The incidence of migraine and headache also reduces in the elderly[20], as stress chemicals are reduced by around 40% after the age of 65.

Women often experience headache and migraine during menstruation. In fact, every musculoskeletal pain is worse during menstruation, as chemicals called prostaglandins are released in that process. Prostaglandins attach to receptors and open up electrical channels in the brain, increasing electrical activity in the pathways that control pain. Females also produce almost

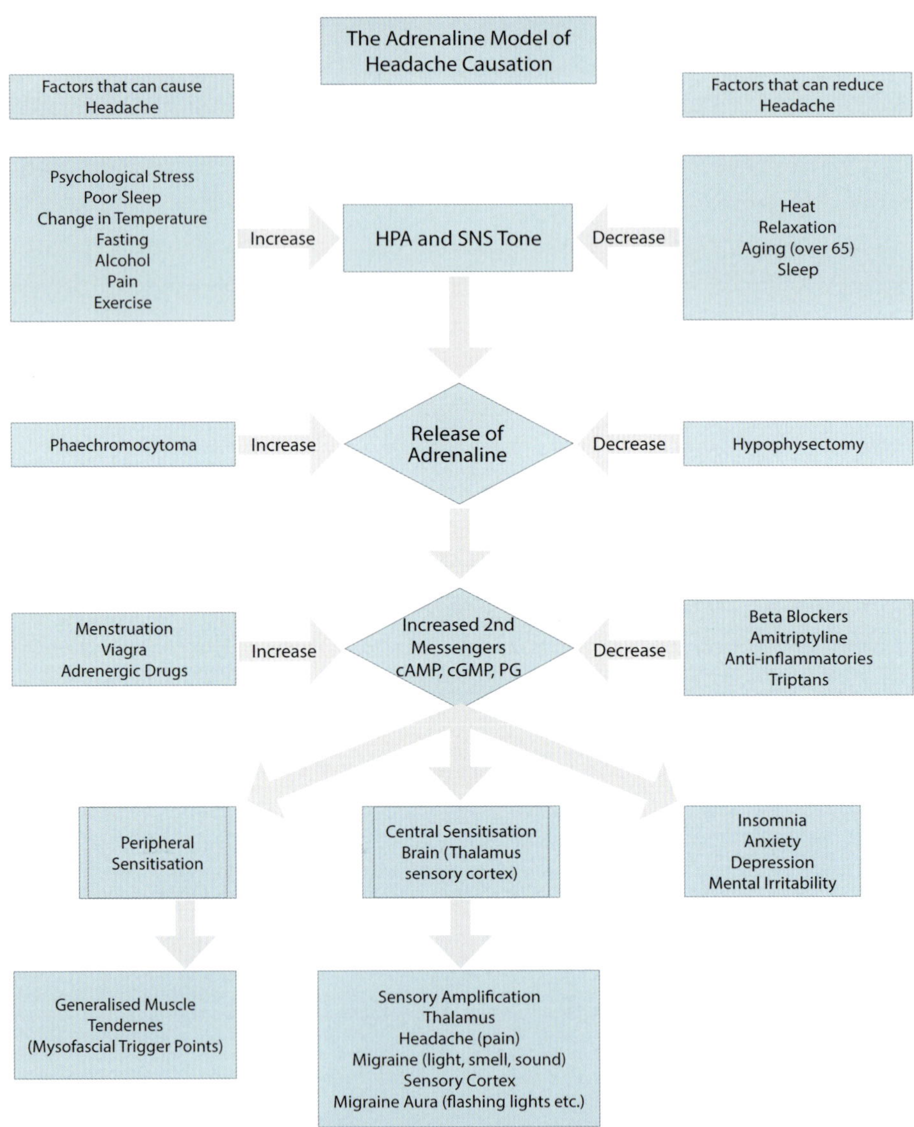

Figure 7.4

The original diagram of the Adrenaline Model of Headache Causation formed during my PhD thesis.

one-third more stress chemicals than males for any given stress. This may also help explain the increased risk of experiencing headache symptoms.

Many headache triggers – including stress, not eating, sleep disturbance, neck pain, alcohol, smoke, sleeping late, food, exercise, and sexual activity – increase both adrenaline and the activity of the stress nervous system. Alcohol causes the release of adrenaline and other stress chemicals in the body, which build up overnight. Electrical channels are opened in the brain, creating headache pain. This explains why we have a hangover. Drinking water helps hangovers probably by diluting and excreting adrenaline rather than through helping dehydration. (This would appear to be confirmed by the fact that headache disorders are uncommon in Africa, where dehydration is extremely common due to the intense heat). A viral illness will also release chemicals in the brain. This increases electrical signals in the pain pathways, often causing generalised body ache.

Research has shown that hand-warming[21], biofeedback[22], meditation[23], exercise[24] and sauna[25] have been effective in reducing headache symptoms. All of these act by reducing the activity of the stress nervous system and are examined in Chapter 8.

CASE STUDY: *Tessa*

Tessa, a 50 year old female, developed neck pain 18 years ago after landing on her head and twisting her neck while on a trampoline. She had experienced a constant headache every day for the past 18 years. She had also experienced an increased frequency of migraines since this accident. Her sleep had been disturbed and she was waking with a headache and neck pain that also radiated into the back of her shoulder.

Over the years Tessa had tried several medications and sought advice from many health professionals to try and find the cause of her symptoms, as well as a cure. She even had an operation to burn the nerves that supply the facet joints in the neck (radiofrequency neurotomy), without any success. When she presented she had a restricted range of motion of her neck, as well as tenderness over nearly all the muscles surrounding her head and neck.

After 18 years of suffering an MRI scan of her neck was performed. This showed dehydration, narrowing and protrusion of two discs in the lower neck, as seen in figure 7.5.

I suggested to Tessa that her neck was likely to be causing her increased headache and migraine symptoms. I advised her how to change postures to reduce the pressure on the lower neck, as well as prescribing a traction collar. She also had some treatment of the muscles surrounding her neck. A few weeks later she was completely free of neck pain and headache for several days, for the first time since the accident, and overall her symptoms have improved.

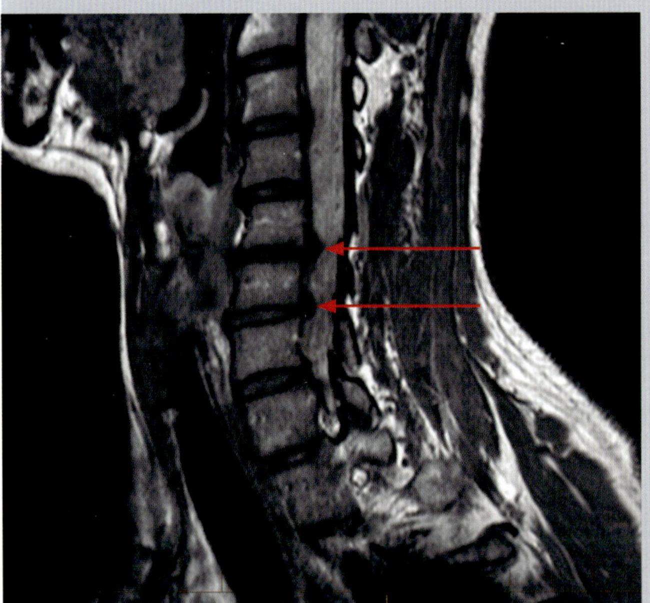

Figure 7.5
The MRI scan shows dehydration, narrowing and protrusion of the two lower discs in the lower neck (as shown by arrows) which were responsible for chronic headache symptoms. The headache symptoms subsided once treatment was directed to the neck.

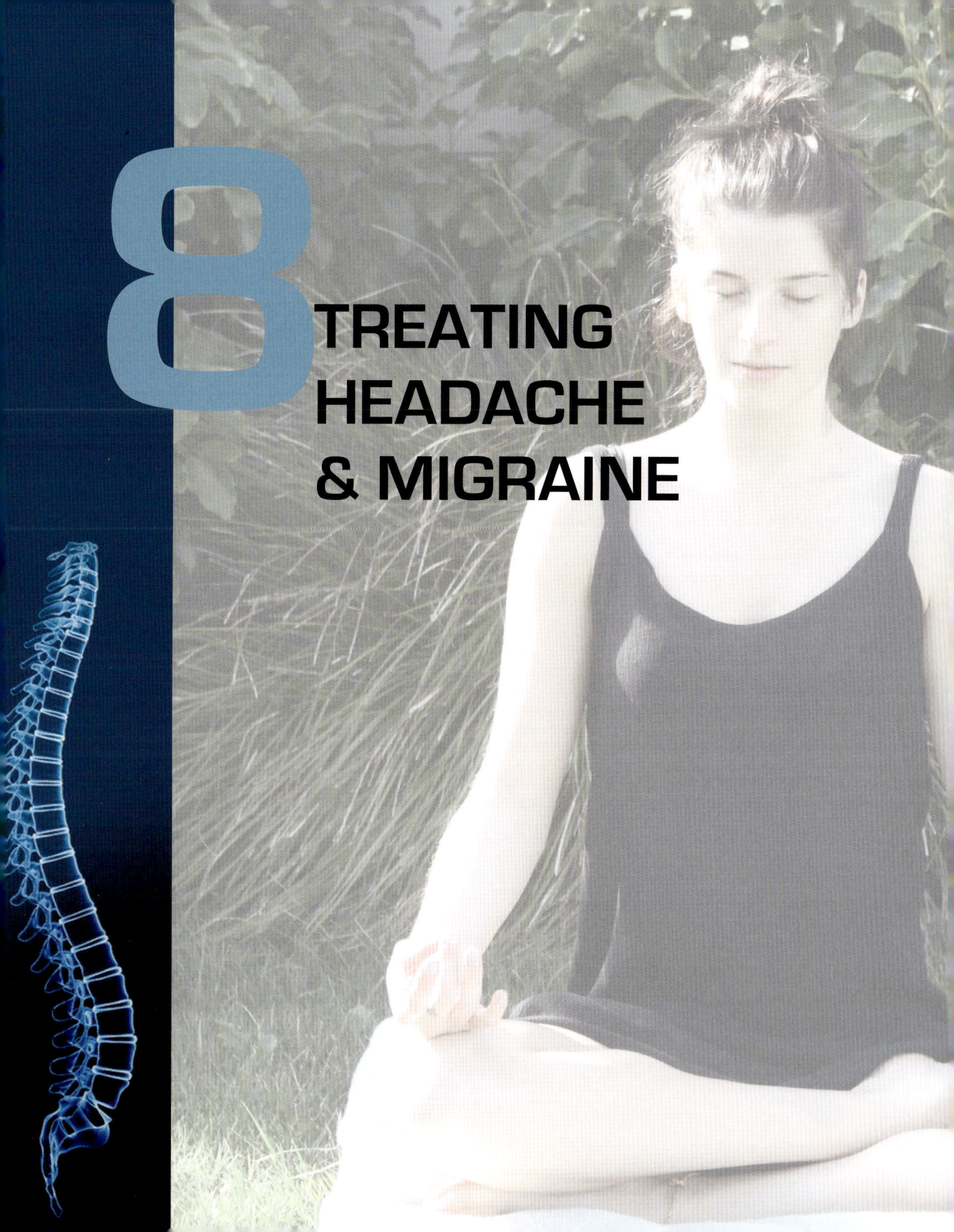

8 TREATING HEADACHE & MIGRAINE

Headache and migraine treatment can be aimed at the pain centres of the brain and spinal cord as well as the neck. Medications attach to receptors and reduce electrical activity in the brain and spinal cord. Reducing stress chemicals will also help reduce electrical activity within the brain pain centre.

Headache medication

Medications for headache and migraine include the use of painkillers (analgesics) for acute episodes of headache. Analgesics include paracetamol, Tylenol, diclofenac, ibuprofen and other commonly taken headache remedies available over the counter. The acute treatment of migraine includes standard analgesics as well as ergotamine, the triptans, and anti-nausea medications or combinations of these.

If the frequency of headache is greater than 10 to 15 days per month, regular medication can be prescribed to prevent headache. Preventative medications include beta-blockers, a range of anti-depressant, anti-epileptic medications as well as calcium channel blockers. Medications that reduce headache and migraine symptoms generally reduce electricity in the pain centres in the brain. Beta-blockers block adrenaline receptors; calcium-channel blockers work by blocking the calcium channels and decreasing their excitability. Amitriptyline, which is the best preventative medication in trials for tension headache, has been shown to change both adrenaline and serotonin levels, reducing stress.

In the last few decades, Botox injections have gained favour for the treatment of headache and migraine in particular. A medical review of Botox injections[26] stated seven medical trials for chronic tension-type headache showed no benefit of Botox injections and three large medical trials for migraine also showed no significant benefit. It seems that Botox is not a panacea for headache or migraine, and remains an expensive option.

Non-medication treatment

Several studies have looked at reducing headache by performing activities known to reduce the activity of the stress nervous system. The trials have tested meditation, heat, regular exercise and sauna.

A medical study of meditation for tension headache[23] which looked at over 300 people, found complete relief of headache in over three quarters of the patients. Depression and anxiety scores also improved.

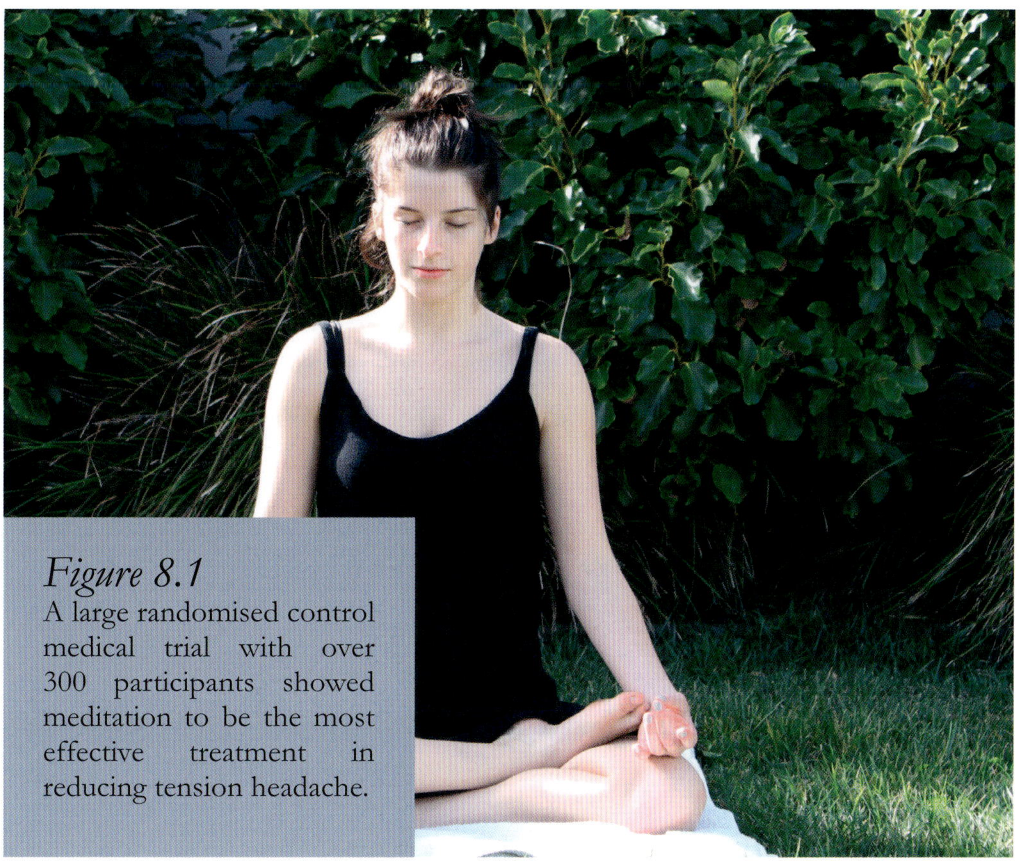

Figure 8.1
A large randomised control medical trial with over 300 participants showed meditation to be the most effective treatment in reducing tension headache.

Headache patients have been shown to have reduced hand temperatures when compared to people without headache[27]. Warming the hands dilates the blood vessels and send signals back to the brain to reduce the production of stress chemicals. Hand warming has been found to help reduce headache symptoms by several researchers[28].

As part of my PhD, I conducted a randomised study using 20-minute sauna sessions three times a week for six weeks on patients with chronic tension-type headache[25]. The patients had experienced 24 out of 28 days headache for

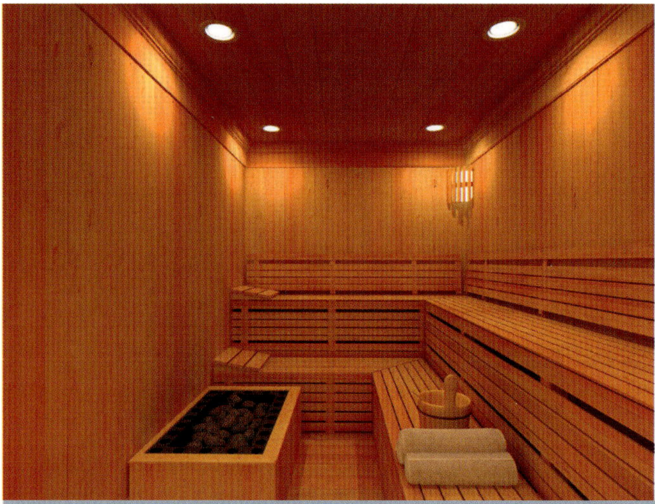

Figure 8.2
A randomised control trial showed the sauna to be effective for people with tension headache.

an average of 16 years. The study showed the sauna group experienced a 45% reduction in headache intensity and a 45% reduction in headache frequency. Half the participants in the sauna group were almost headache-free at the end of the trial. In a telephone survey performed 12 months after the trial, the people who had seen improvements were still headache-free.

Regular exercise to where the heart races, can reduce stress chemicals. Medical studies on both headache[29] and migraine have shown exercise can reduce the intensity of headache and frequency of migraine. When compared to exercise, one of the latest migraine prevention tablets was found to be no better than exercising three times a week[24].

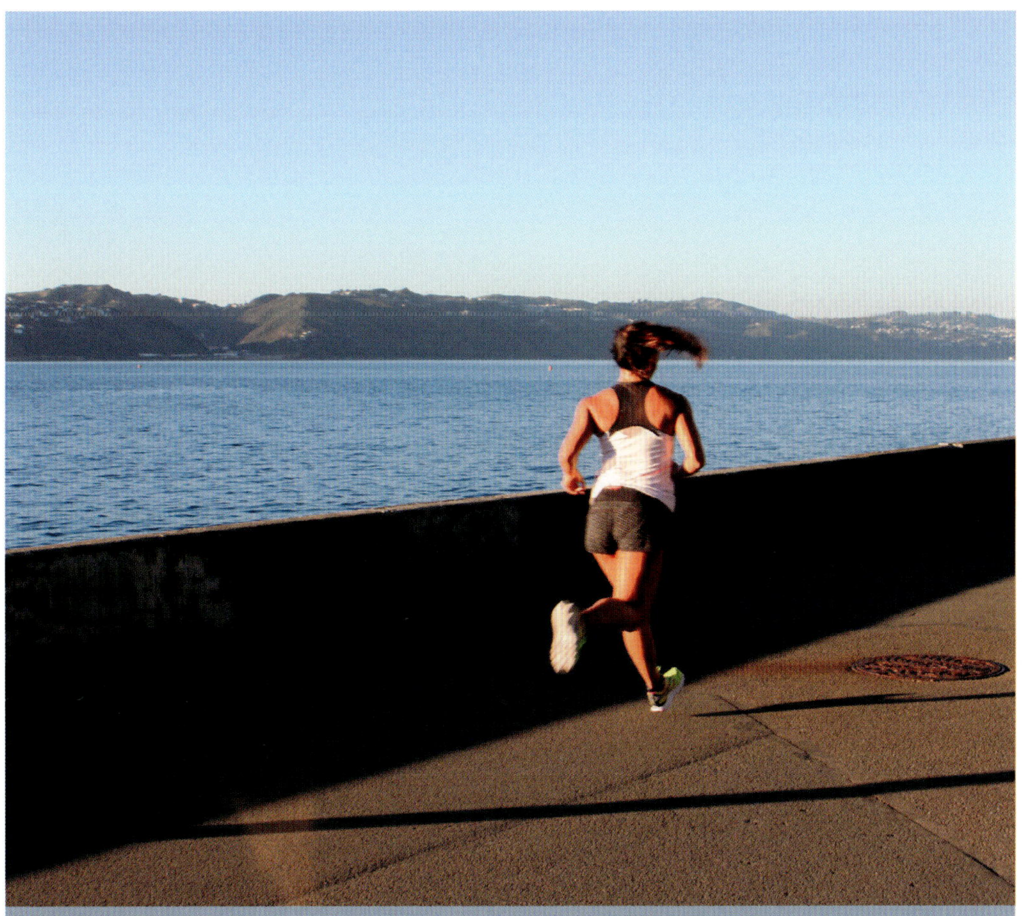

Figure 8.3
A randomised control trial showed exercise three times a week to be as effective as the best available migraine preventative treatment.

The role of the neck in headache and migraine

How does the neck play a part in headache and migraine? The neck is the most common source of pain in people who experience headache. Head scans are the most common investigations for people experiencing headache and migraine symptoms, but 99% of the time they are within normal limits as the head is the not source of pain, but rather the site where pain is experienced. Pain arising from the neck is often experienced as a headache due to pain spreading into the head (referred pain).

Any structure in the neck such as the disc, ligaments, facet joints or muscles can refer pain into the head by the spread of electrical signals in the brain. A good example of referred pain from the neck is seen by the pattern of pain from neck muscle knots.

The muscle knots (myofascial trigger points) cause pain when stimulated. The pain from muscle knots can then spread as seen in Chapter 3; this process has been the subject of multiple books that map the pain patterns of various muscles.

In summary, when treating patients with headache and migraine, it is worth looking at the neck as a source of pain. A proportion of headaches may be due to stress chemicals in the brain turning on the pain switch (hangover headache, pure tension headache) but most are a combination of pain sensitivity of the brain and the neck. Treatment targeting the brain to reduce pain sensitivity, as well as the neck, will together often provide longer-term relief.

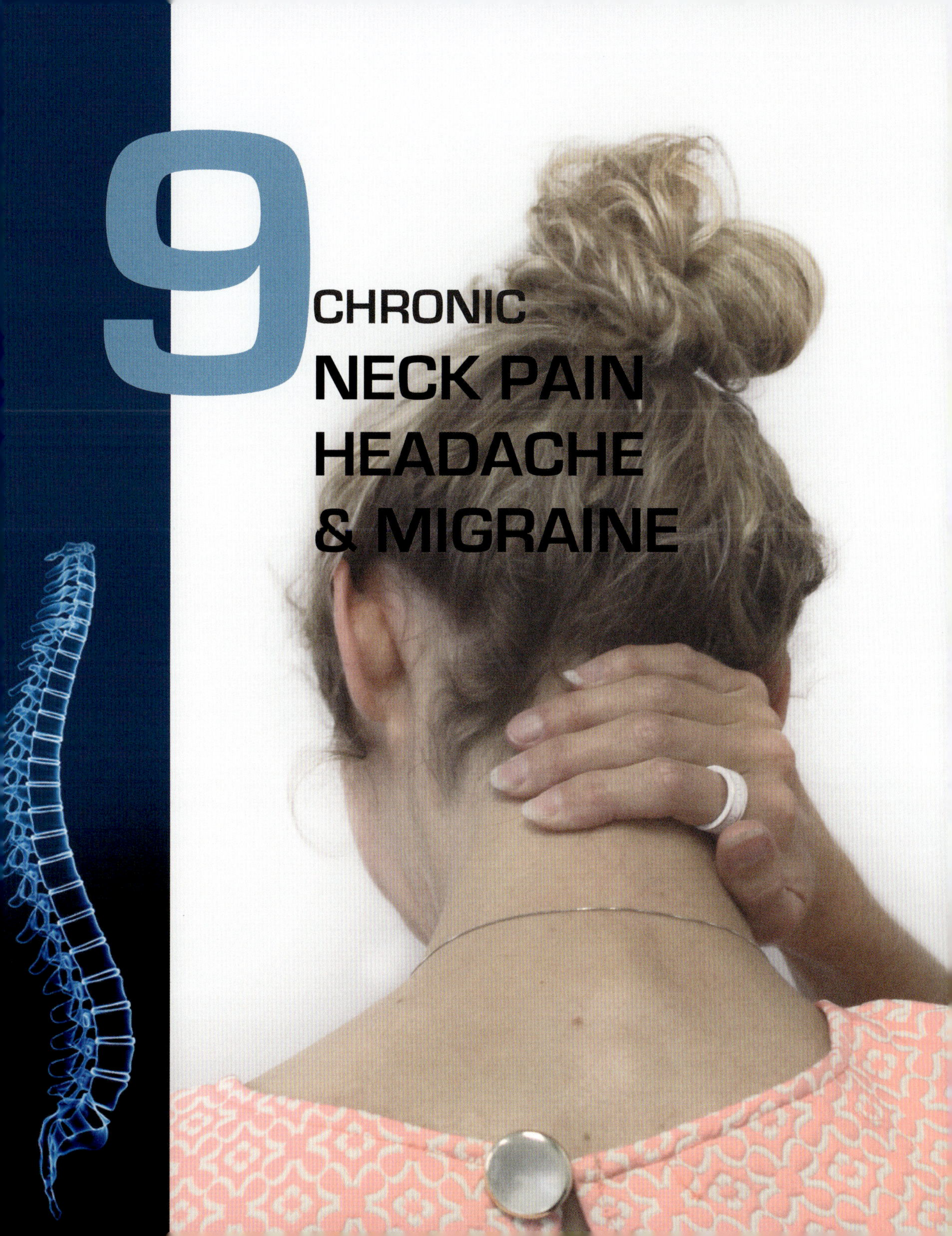

9 CHRONIC NECK PAIN HEADACHE & MIGRAINE

The Adrenaline Nightmare

Fortunately, most people with neck pain and headache find that their condition improves and they can return to their normal activities. Around 5% of sufferers, however, continue to experience neck pain and headache on a daily basis and become limited in their activities. After many years of observing chronic pain patients, I have noticed that living with pain often leads to stress-related conditions such as insomnia, anxiety and depression. Moreover, the risk increases with the number of episodes of neck pain experienced. So why do people with long-term pain develop stress-related symptoms? I decided to investigate this question as part of my PhD, hoping that understanding how these problems develop could lead to solutions for them.

The answer, I discovered, lies in stress chemicals that are released when a patient experiences pain. Adrenaline is the major stress chemical released, and I called the development of these symptoms the "Adrenaline Nightmare". Cold, psychological stress, hunger, excess alcohol, poor sleep, and viral illness along with pain can all activate the stress pathways, release adrenaline into the body and brain and perpetuate the Adrenaline Nightmare. Other stress chemicals released in the brain and spinal cord include histamine, serotonin and noradrenaline.

These stress chemicals attach to the brain pain switch, increasing electricity and amplifying pain. When pain amplifies, it can spread to other regions of the body and result in widespread pain, often called fibromyalgia. Furthermore, the stress associated with not being able to work, dealing with insurance companies for compensation, relationship difficulties, and loss of self-esteem can add to the release of stress chemicals and perpetuate pain. Life events such as bereavement and separation also increase stress chemicals.

The alcohol hangover

Excess alcohol activates the stress nervous system and leads to the release of

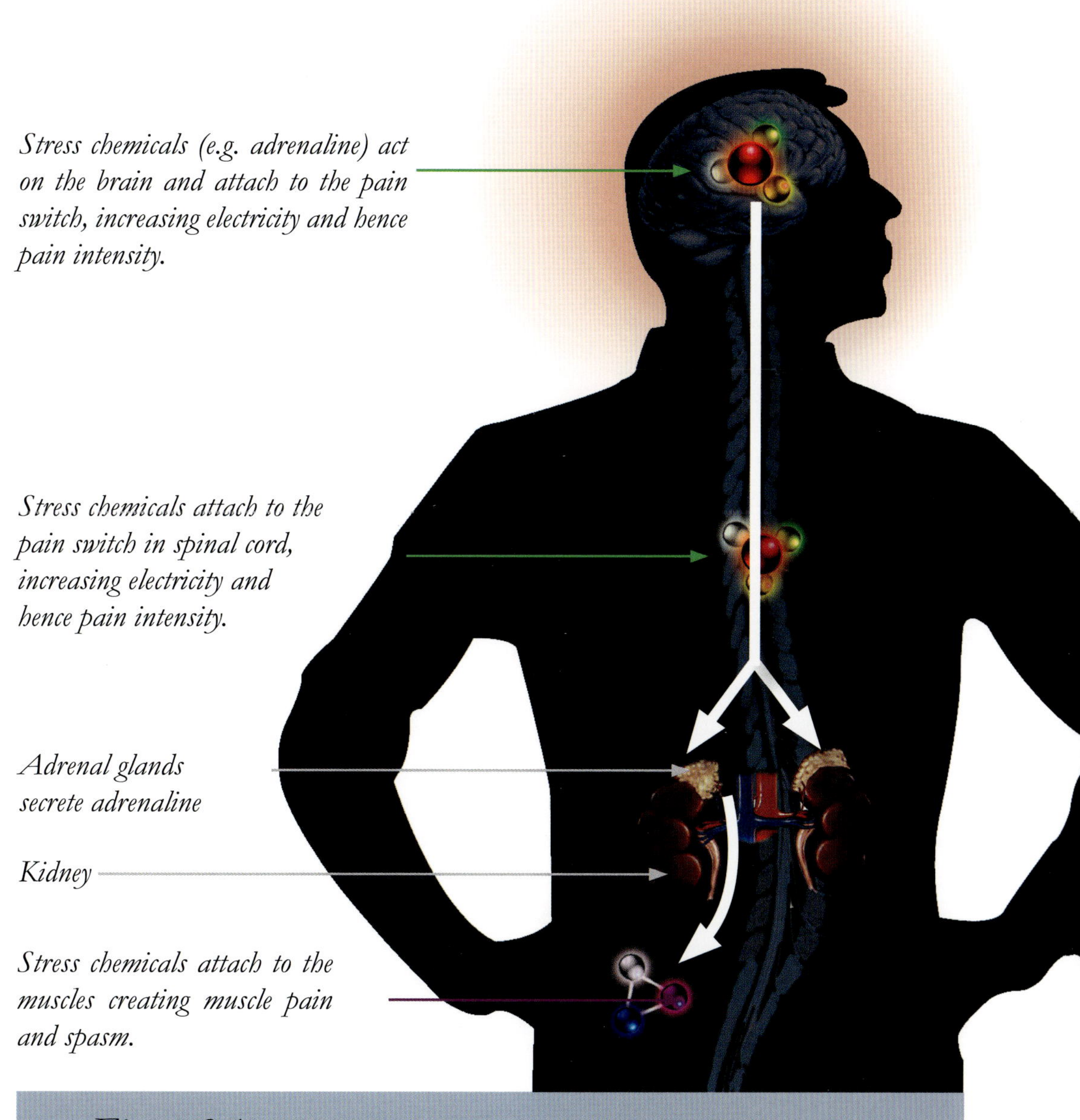

Figure 9.1

Stress chemicals act in the brain and body leading to increased pain and muscle spasm.

stress chemicals. Overnight, the body releases adrenaline which increases the electricity in the pain switches in the brain, causing you to wake with headache or even whole body ache in the morning. People often attribute hangover headache to dehydration, but this is unlikely as people in Africa, a part of the world where dehydration is prevalent, suffer very few headaches. Drinking water does however help hangover headache as you flush the adrenaline out of the bloodstream by increasing the urinary excretion of adrenaline.

The fight/flight response

The release of stress chemicals activates the fight/flight response in the body, a very primitive response designed primarily to escape danger. Stress chemicals prepare the body for vigorous physical activity and are depleted by running or fighting. Unfortunately, when released by pain or stress, stress chemicals are not consumed and therefore build up in the brain. Stress chemicals can keep people alert, awake, on edge and anxious. This feeling can disturb sleep and cause people to wake at night due to the smallest disturbance. If stress chemicals continue to build up in the brain, individuals can even develop panic attacks or depression.

Adrenaline, in particular, increases blood flow to the muscles up to 10 times for running and fighting, sharpens the eyesight and hearing, and reduces blood flow to all the non-emergency organs in the body. To supply the muscles with increased blood flow, the heart must pump vigorously, often resulting in palpitations (an awareness of heart beat) and increased blood pressure. Adrenaline reduces blood flow to the skin and switches off skin repair cells, leading to dry skin. Blood flow is reduced to the extremities, causing cold hands and feet (often called Raynaud's phenomena), a sign of an overactive stress nervous system.

The digestive system is not essential when you are faced with a life-threatening situation, so adrenaline release can lead to a 40% reduction in blood flow to the gut. Digestive enzymes and movement of the gut are also reduced, leading to irritable bowel syndrome. Stress also leads to the development of stomach ulcers.

Glucose and fats are released to provide fuel for the vigorous physical activity required while escaping danger. However, when adrenaline is released purely for pain, glucose and fat are not consumed by vigorous physical activity and can aggravate diabetes and heart disease. Furthermore, stress chemicals constrict the blood vessels of the body and increase blood pressure. Raised glucose and fats in the blood stream, combined with increased blood pressure, are the principal reasons that stress is the major cause of heart disease worldwide.

Depleting stress chemicals

When treating patients with long-term pain, it is essential to advise them how to manage their stress response. Managing the factors that increase stress chemicals, such as excess alcohol, poor sleep, psychological stressors and reducing pain, are essential in achieving a long-term successful result. Having a calm mind is very helpful, as it makes the individual less reactive to the environment and the potentially stressful events that occur in daily life, reducing the build-up of stress chemicals. Adding therapies to reduce stress chemicals, such as heat, exercise and relaxation, can also help reduce pain and stress-related conditions.

How can you prevent the build-up of stress chemicals? Reducing stress chemicals in the circulation will help the distress and insomnia that patients often develop from chronic pain.

First, the stressors that are present must be addressed. These include an individual's relationship, work situation, financial position, pain, and poor sleep, among many others. Sometimes you need to stand back, as if observing your life from a distance, and examine how you can reduce the stressors around you. You may need to seek the advice of a friend or professional therapist to achieve this.

Next, it is worthwhile looking at how you respond to the environment and to events. Do you catastrophise and think about the worst thing that could possibly happen? Do you continue to analyse past events over and over again?

CASE STUDY: *Sue*

Sue presented with a diagnosis of fibromyalgia, having experienced pain throughout her body over the past 30 years. She arrived on several medications including Omeprazole, Quetiapine, cholecalciferol, calcium carbonate, Paroxetine, naprosyn, DHC Continuus and Tramadol. Sue did not know what was causing her symptoms, but while recounting her pain history she told me about an accident in which she rode her bike straight into a pole and landed heavily on the ground.

After education on the effects of stress chemicals, Sue attended the sauna and swimming pool, and over several months her pain settled into her neck and low back. MRI scans of her neck (Figure 9.2) and low back (Figure 9.3) were performed and showed damaged discs to be the likely source of her symptoms. With time and increasing intensity her pain had spread to her head, arms, chest, low back and legs. After the source of her pain had been located, treatment was aimed at the neck and low back, with an improvement of her symptoms. She was very pleased to have a diagnosis of why she experienced so much pain.

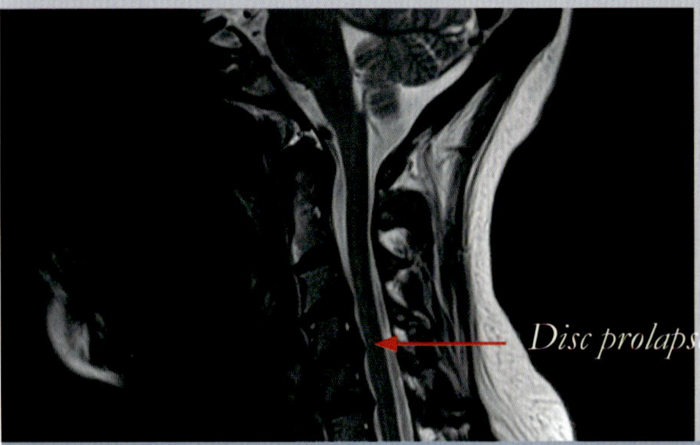

Figure 9.2
The MRI scan showed a straight neck as well as a disc prolapse between the fourth and fifth vertebrae in the neck.

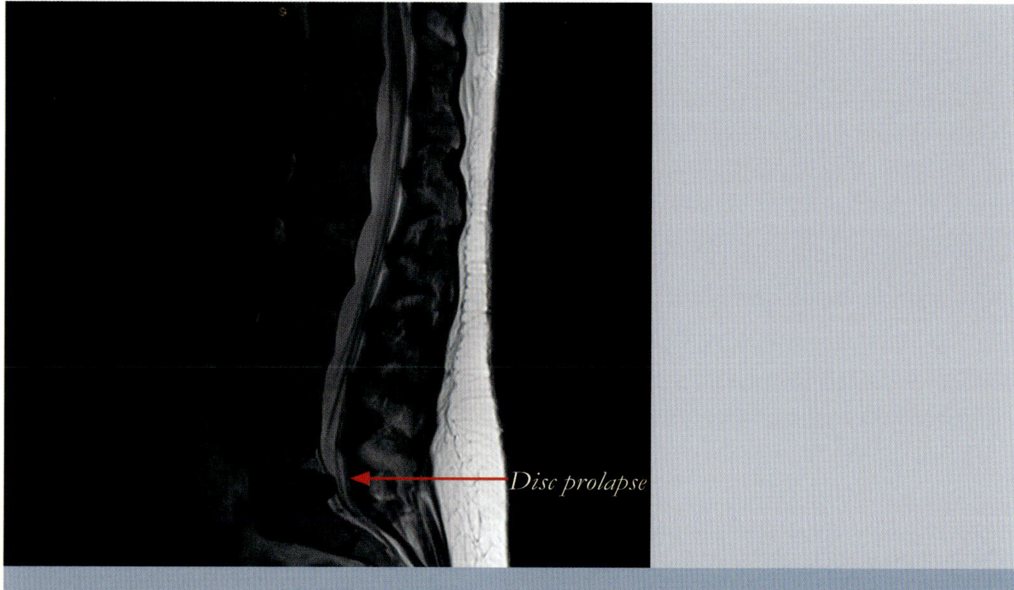

Figure 9.3
The MRI scan shows a lumbar spine disc prolapse and narrowing at the lowest disc of the lumbar spine.

When adverse events occur, some people will brush them off as being minor and no threat to their lives, while others make a big deal out of them. If you can brush them off, you will release fewer stress chemicals. But if you catastrophise, you will flood your brain and body with stress chemicals, perpetuating the Adrenaline Nightmare. It is worthwhile practising meditation, yoga, or tai chi to calm the mind. Learning mindfulness, or other techniques to help your mind process your environment and events that occur, will help ensure you cope better with what goes on around you.

Techniques to burn stress chemicals include regular exercise and heat. I recommend that patients exercise for 30 minutes at least four times a week to help them return to a normal life. Exercise can be performed in two bursts of 15 minutes if fatigue is a problem. Exercise such as walking does not deplete the build-up of stress chemicals, so more rigorous exercise needs to be performed.

Heat reduces the activity of the stress nervous system. Normally the activation of the stress nervous system constricts the blood vessels in the skin, but heat causes these blood vessels to dilate. When the skin's blood vessels dilate, a signal is sent to the brain to tell it to stop producing stress chemicals such as adrenaline. The deep relaxation felt after a sauna is due to this reduction in the activity of the stress nervous system.

A clinical trial[25] performed, as part of my PhD, on people suffering daily headache showed the severity and duration of headache reduced on average over 40% after they attended the sauna for 20 minutes three times a week for six weeks. The improvements were sustained for a year after the trial finished. If you can tolerate heat, this is an excellent way to reset your stress pathways without using medication. If you cannot stand the heat for long, after five to 10 minutes you can leave the sauna, have a warm shower, then reduce the temperature to cold. This will reset your temperature switch and allow you to get back in the sauna. Remember to drink plenty of water. Other options include hot baths and spa pools, although these do not provide the same intense heat as a sauna.

Breathing exercises also work in the same way as heat by signalling the stress nervous system to relax. Instead of breathing by expanding the chest, you need to learn to breathe by moving the abdominal muscles. This results in deeper and slower breaths that reduce the activity of the stress nervous system. Deep relaxation or meditation reduces the activity of the stress nervous system and subsequent production of stress chemicals. In one large study, 20 minutes of meditation per day helped reduce headaches by 95%. Any relaxation therapy may help if performed for 20 minutes daily.

Sleep disturbance and fatigue

Sleep disturbance creates fatigue by upsetting the pattern of cortisol release. Cortisol is another chemical released during stress. It also has a daily release pattern that is important in maintaining energy. Cortisol levels can

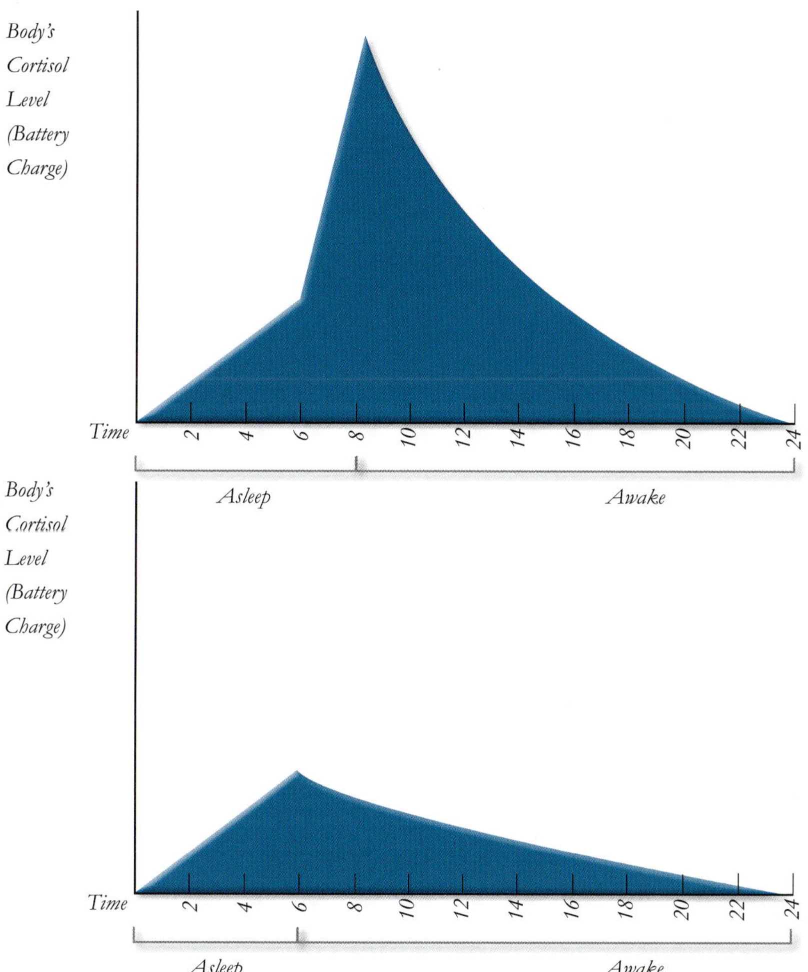

Figure 9.4

The top graph shows the normal patterns of cortisol secretion. The highest levels are present in the morning and give you energy. If you sleep less than four to six hours, you may wake without the cortisol levels reaching their peak, as shown in the second graph.

be thought of as an indicator of your battery charge, with high levels in the morning, giving rise to feeling like a "box of birds", and low levels in the evening, leading to tiredness. Cortisol increases overnight, with a slow steady rise in the first six hours of sleep, followed by a rapid rise in the last few hours (Figure 9.4). When you wake the battery is fully charged. If you wake before you have slept for six hours, your levels of cortisol are likely to be sub-optimal and you will feel tired. Over many months of poor sleep, the production of cortisol loses its pattern, and after several years the level of cortisol is often depleted as the gland suffers burnout (commonly called adrenal fatigue).

The pattern of cortisol release can be best understood by looking at jetlag. Jetlag occurs due to a mismatch between your cortisol levels and your time zone. If you travel halfway around the world, your battery will be fully charged at night instead of in the morning. You feel energy at night and are tired in the morning. Over a week or so, you adjust to your new time zone as your cortisol levels change.

Sometimes it is difficult to restore a sleep pattern. Medications may be useful in the short term by helping to restore a sleep pattern that leads to improved energy and allows you to exercise. If you are taking sleeping tablets such as diazepam, temazepam or zopiclone then it is wise to take these no more than three times a week. If taken every day, they stop working as the brain gets used to the tablet, and addiction can occur.

Other sedatives including amitriptyline, Tegretol and quetiapine belong to a range of tablets that are used for epilepsy, depression and psychosis. One of the main benefits of these tablets is that they all cause sleepiness, as they act on receptors that cause sedation. They can be taken daily, and trial and error will determine which suits you best and causes the fewest side effects. Some people may be intolerant of certain medications. If you cannot tolerate one tablet, try another until you find one that suits you.

Tablets can be a useful addition to more natural remedies such as going to a sauna, especially in the short term to improve sleep. In patients with chronic sleep deprivation and fatigue where the adrenal gland has stopped producing cortisol (adrenal fatigue), the gland has lost the ability to restore its normal pattern of cortisol production and thus restore energy. Sleeping well for seven to eight hours per night for several months is required for the adrenal gland to start functioning again and let the individual wake feeling refreshed. Ensuring minimal sleep disturbance from noise, as well as avoiding caffeinated drinks or stimulating activity late at night, are important factors in ensuring a good night's sleep.

Conclusion

Neck pain, headache and migraine are often difficult to understand for those who do not suffer from them. There are no visible signs such as a plaster cast or deformity for your suffering – it is essentially invisible. Often patients do not mention their problem to others, including health professionals, due to the lack of solutions.

For the health professionals who treat neck pain, it is best to give advice on disc pain, as this is the most common source of neck pain. Information on the structure and function of the disc, postures to reduce disc pressure and avoiding activities or postures that increase disc pressure are all beneficial for the patient. Tablets can be prescribed to help reduce pain and to help sleep, if sleep is disturbed.

Patients appreciate learning the cause of their neck pain and the management strategies that can be aimed at the cause of symptoms. If a patient's pain does not subside or recurs frequently, it is essential to find the cause of their symptoms in order to understand how to deal with their symptoms. An X-ray may help if neck pain has been present for many years; otherwise an MRI scan is the best test to show the disc structure. Tests must be correlated with the pain story and examination findings to ensure that what is found on the tests matches up with the symptoms.

Once the patient knows what is causing their pain, they can adopt activities and/or postures that will lessen pain, and discard activities and/or postures that aggravate it.

I worked on this book over a two-year period and have tested the management strategies described with hundreds of neck pain, headache and migraine patients over seven years. Some patients had been in pain for just a few months, others for more than 20 years. Many patients improved substantially by simply using traction, heat, exercising regularly, changing postures to reduce pressure on the neck discs and having their muscles treated. This has allowed them to reduce dependence on healthcare providers as well as stop taking medications. Patients that did not respond to these simple measures required further investigations to identify the cause of their symptoms and appropriate management strategies to give them relief.

If you suffer from neck pain, headache or migraine, I hope this book helps you understand and manage your pain.

Glossary

aberration Deviation from the normal or expected.

acupuncture Procedure adapted from traditional chinese medicine in which fine needles are placed into the skin and muscles for therapeutic purposes and pain relief.

adrenaline Stress chemical released from the adrenal glands when the body is under stress.

anaesthetic /local anaesthetic Agent injected into an area of the body to numb it or take away sensation.

analgesia Medication that acts to relieve pain.

annular ligament/annulus fibrosis/ring ligament Tough circular ligament surrounding the soft core of an intervertebral disc.

annular tear Tear or hole in the outer disc wall of an intervertbral disc.

bone scan Nuclear scanning test that finds areas of increased bone turnover.

cartilage Flexible and tough connective tissue comprised mostly of water that cushions joints; significant portion of intervetebral discs.

chronic pain Pain lasting for longer than three months.

complex regional pain syndrome/regional sympathetic dystrophy Pain usually in an arm or a leg that is more severe than expected for that injury. It can be due to a nerve injury and touch is painful.

congenital abnormality Defect or variation present at birth.

CT scan Computed Tomography scan where multiple X-rays are taken and used to form a cross-sectional picture of the area.

degenerative change Progressive narrowing of the cartilage in joints and the discs in the spine with secondary osteophytes (bony spurs)

dermatome An area of skin mainly supplied by a single spinal nerve.

diagnosis Nature or cause of a disease or injury.

disc Shock absorber (washer) in between the bones of the spine.

discectomy Surgical removal of a herniated or protruding disc.

disc bulge Small protrusion of a disc seen on an MRI scan.

disc prolapse Condition in which the disc no longer sits within its normal confines and the gel centre of the disc squeezes through the ring ligament.

disc replacement Artificial implant used in place of a disc.

electrical therapies Use of electrical energy as a medical treatment.

endplate Surface of the vertebra that comes into contact with the disc.

facet joint/zygoapophyseal joint Synovial joint that helps support the weight of the body and controls movement between individual vertebrae of the spine.

fluoroscopy A method that provides real time X-ray imaging; especially useful for guiding diagnostic and interventional procedures.

fusion Surgical technique that joins two or more vertebrae together to stop them from moving.

foraminotomy An operation used to relieve pressure on nerves that are being compressed by the passages within the bones of the vertebrae. Literally, cutting a hole in the bone.

genetic predisposition Having the genes that make a condition more likely to occur.

hard tissues Mineralised tissues like bone and cartilage.

headache Pain anywhere in the region of the head. It can be a symptom of a number of conditions of the head or the neck.

insomnia Difficulty getting to sleep or staying asleep.

invasive treatment Treatment that involves entering the body.

laminectomy Surgical removal of the lamina (bone that sits at the back of the spinal cord) to increase space for the spinal cord.

ligament Band of fibrous tissue connecting two bones together.

lordosis The inward (concave) curvature of the cervical and lumbar spines.

lumbar spine/lower back Refers to the lowest five segments in the spine.

manual therapy Hands-on treatment, for example: massage, mobilisation and manipulation.

migraine Hereditary predisposition to sensory amplification (light, sound, touch, pain and smell). Most commonly associated with severe headache characterised by sharp pain that usually affects one side of the head. The headache is often accompanied by nausea, vomiting, and visual disturbances.

manipulation Manual therapy which employs thrust techniques to stretch joints.

memory foam Polyurethane with chemicals which increase its viscosity, providing support, especially for the spine. Commonly used for beds and pillows.

mobilisation Process intended to make a joint mobile by gentle forces.

MRI scan Magnetic Resonance Imaging produces high quality images of soft tissues such as the disc in the spine using magnetic technology.

musculoskeletal medicine Medicine for both acute and chronic conditions of the musculoskeletal system, i.e. muscle, joints, nerves, ligaments, cartilage and spinal discs.

pain Sensory and emotional experience that creates physical and psychological suffering.

pain pathway Route along which pain signals are sent to the brain.

pain switch Relay switch in the brain or spinal cord that conducts pain.

prolotherapy Injection therapy used to treat various types of chronic pain.

psychiatrist Doctor who specialises in the diagnosis and treatment of mental health disorders.

psychologist Professional who studies the mind and looks at behaviour, cognition and social influences.

radiculopathy Condition affecting the nerve root. Pressure on the nerve root causes pain, numbness, weakness and pins and needles.

radiofrequency neurotomy A procedure to reduce back and neck pain, using heat generated by radio waves to damage specific nerves causing the pain.

randomised control trial A scientific experiment where people selected randomly are allocated one or the other of the different treatments under the study. The random control is the gold standard for clinical trials.

receptor Group of nerve endings that responds to stimuli.

referred pain Pain felt at a site other than that where the pain originated.

sacro-iliac joint Joint in the bony pelvis between the sacrum and the ilium of the pelvic girdle, where they meet on either side of the lower back.

saline Salt solution.

side effects Undesirable effect of a drug or therapy.

soft tissues Tissues that connect, support or surround other tissues or organs, and are not made of bone, e.g. muscles, ligaments and tendons.

steroids Group of synthetic hormones that promote the growth and healing of tissue.

stress chemicals Chemicals like adrenaline that are released into the blood stream when the body is stressed or in pain.

sympathetic nervous system/stress nervous system The nervous system in the body that detects changes (stress), such as heat, cold and psychological stress, causing the release of stress chemicals.

tendon Fibrous tissue that connects muscle to bone.

traction A mechanism for relieving pressure on the spine, e.g cervical collar.

vertebrae Bony segments that form the spine.

X-rays Electromagnetic radiation that is used to take pictures of the bones in the body.

References

1. Jonsson H, Bring G, Rauschning W, et al. Hidden cervical spine injuries in traffic accident victims with skull fractures. J Spinal Disorders 1991: 4, 251-263.

2. Kanji, G. Convergent referred pain mechanisms: the research and implications for clinical practice. Australasian Musculoskeletal Medicine 2005: 10(2), 124-126.

3. Cloward, RB. Cervical discography: A contribution to the aetiology and mechanism of neck, shoulder and arm pain. Annals of Surgery 1959: 150(60), 1052-1064.

4. Kuijper, B, Tans, J, Beelen, A, Nollet, F, de Visser, M. Cervical collar or physiotherapy versus wait and see policy for recent onset cervical radiculopathy: randomised trial. British Medical Journal 2009:339:b3883.

5. Braf, MM and Rosner, S. Chronic headache: A study of over 2000 cases. New York State Journal of Medicine 1960: 60, 3987-3994.

6. Lee, M, Wong, F, Tang, FT, Chang, WH and Chiou, WK. Design and assessment of an adaptive intermittent cervical traction modality with EMG biofeedback. Biomechanical Engineering 1996: 118(4), 597-600.

7. Olivero, W, Dulebohn, S. Results of halter cervical traction for the treatment of cervical radiculopathy: retrospective review of 81 patients. Neurosurgical Focus 2002: 12(2), 1-4.

8. Chung, TS, Lee, YJ, Kang, SW, Park, CJ, Kang, WS, Shim, YW. Reducibility of cervical disk herniation: evaluation at MR imaging during cervical traction with a nonmagnetic traction device. Radiology 2002: 225(3), 895-900.

9. Shealy, CN. IRB approved MRI study of the effects of Axial Linear Traction and expanding ellipsoidal decompression via posture pump on cervical curve, disc protrusions and disc height. 2008.

10. Moffet, JAK, Hughes, GI, Griffiths, P. An investigation of the effects of cervical traction. Part 1: Clinical effectiveness. Clinical rehabilitation 1990; 4, 205-211.

11. Zylbergold, RS, and Piper, MC. Cervical spine disorders - A comparison of three types of traction. Spine 1985: 10, 867-871.

12. Ylinen, J, Takala E, Nyaken M, Hakkinen A, Malkia E, Pohojolainen T, Karppi, S, Kautiainen H, Airaksinen, O. Active neck muscle training in the treatment of chronic neck pain in women: A randomised controlled trial. Journal of the American Medical Association 2003: 289 (19), 2509-16.
13. Yelland, MJ, Glasziou, PP, Bogduk, N, Schluter, PJ, McKernon, M. Prolotherapy injections, saline injections and exercises for chronic low back pain: a randomised trial. Spine 2004: 29(1), 9–16.
14. Kanji, G. 2006 The management of lumbar spine pain. Australasian Musculoskeletal Journal, 11(2): 91-97.
15. Matsumoto M, Okada, E, Ichihara, D, Watanabe, K, Chiba, K, Toyama, Y, Fujiwara, H, Momoshima, S, Nishiwaki, Y, Iwanami, A, Ikegami, T, Takahata, T, Hashimoto, T. Anterior cervical decompression and fusion accelerates adjacent segment degeneration: comparison with asymptomatic volunteers in a ten-year magnetic resonance imaging follow-up study. Spine 2010: 35(1), 36-43.
16. Le, H, Tfelt-Hansen, P, Russell, MB, Skytthe, A, Kyvik, KO and Olesen, J. Co-morbidity of migraine with somatic disease in a large population-based study. Cephalalgia 2010: June 2.
17. Kelman, L. The triggers or precipitants of the acute migraine attack. Cephalalgia 2007: 27, 394-402.
18. Gori, S, Morelli, N, Bellini, G, Bonanni, E, Manca, L, Orlandi, G, et al. Rizatrapine does not change cerebral blood flow velocity during migraine attacks. Brain Research Bulletin 2005: 65(4), 297-300.
19. Schoonman, G, van der Grond, J, Kortmann, C, van der Geest, R., Terwindt, G, Ferrari MD. Migraine headache is not associated with cerebral or meningeal vasodilatation--a 3T magnetic resonance angiography study. Brain. 2008 Aug;131(Pt 8):2192-200.
20. Boardman, H., Thomas, E., Croft, P., & Millson, D. Epidemiology of headache in an English district. Cephalalgia 2003: 23, 129-137.
21. Andrasik, F, Blanchard, EB, Neff, DF, & Rodichok, LD. Biofeedback and relaxation training for chronic headache: A controlled comparison of booster treatments and regular contacts for long-term maintenance. Journal

of Consulting and Clinical Psychology 1984: 52, 609–615.

22. Holroyd, KA, Penzien, DB. Pharmacological versus non-pharmacological prophylaxis of recurrent migraine headache: a meta-analytic review of clinical trials. Pain 1990: 42, Issue 1, 1–13.

23. Kiran, U, Behari, M, Venugopal, P, Vivehanandhan, S, & Pandy, R. The effect of autogenic relaxation on chronic tension headache and in modulating cortisol response. Indian Journal Anesthesia 2005: 49(6), 474-478.

24. Varkey, E, Cider, A, Carlsson, J, & Linde, M. Exercise as migraine prophylaxis: a randomised study using relaxation and topirimate as controls. Cephalalgia 2011: 0(0), 1-11.

25. Kanji, G, Weatherall, M, Peter, R, Purdie, G, Page, R. Efficacy of Regular Sauna Bathing for Chronic Tension-Type Headache: A Randomized Controlled Study. The Journal of Alternative and Complementary Medicine. February 2015, 21(2): 103-109.

26. Schulte-Mattler W, Martinez-Castrillo J. Botulinum toxin therapy of migraine and tension-type headache: comparing different botulinum toxin preparations. European Journal of Neurology 2006: 13 Suppl 1, 51-4.

27. Blanchard, E, Morrill, B, Wittrock, D, Scharff, L, & Jaccard, J. Hand temperature norms for headache, hypertension, and irritable bowel syndrome. Biofeedback and Self Regulation 1989: 14(4), 319-331.

28. Nestoriuc, Y, Martin, A, Rief, W, & Andrasik, F. Biofeedback treatment for headache disorders: A comprehensive efficacy review. Applied Psychophysiology and Biofeedback 2008: 33, 125-140.

29. Narin, S, & Pinar, S. The effects of exercise and exercise-related changes in blood nitric oxide level on migraine headache. Clinical Rehabilitation 2003: 17, 624-630.

Index

Acknowledgements

Thanks to everyone who helped in shaping this book. Preehya Patel, Selena Henry and Sejal Bhikha who worked on the artwork.

Annemaree Naylor, Janene Bone, Dr Clare McMahon, Katherine Barcham, Anthony Davies, John Rietveld and others who read the book and provided valuable feedback. Thanks to Max Rashbrooke for editing the book. Thanks to Mary Varnham for her initial input into a very early version of a manuscript of a book on chronic pain. Thanks goes to all the patients who were instrumental in helping me understand pain and gain insights that have lead to the writing of this book.

Dr Giresh Kanji (Wellington)
April 2015